AYURVEDA FOR BEGINNERS

A Complete Guide to Understanding
and Embracing Ancient Wisdom for
Modern Well-Being and Balance

MONIKA DANIEL

© Copyright 2024 - All rights reserved. The contents of this book may not be reproduced, duplicated or transmitted without direct written permission from the author. Under no circumstances will any legal responsibility or blame be held against the publisher for any reparation, damages, or monetary loss due to the information herein, either directly or indirectly.

Legal Notice: This book is copyright protected. This is only for personal use. You cannot amend, distribute, sell, use, quote or paraphrase any part or the content within this book without the consent of the author.

Disclaimer Notice: Please note the information contained within this document is for educational and entertainment purposes only. Every attempt has been made to provide accurate, up to date and reliable complete information. No warranties of any kind are expressed or implied. Readers acknowledge that the author is not engaging in the rendering of legal, financial, medical or professional advice. The content of this book has been derived from various sources. Please consult a licensed professional before attempting any techniques outlined in this book. By reading this document, the reader agrees that under no circumstances is the author responsible for any losses, direct or indirect, which are incurred as a result of the use of information contained within this document, including, but not limited to, errors, omissions, or inaccuracies.

Table of Contents

Chapter 1: Introduction to Ayurveda 1

    Philosophical Foundations: The Core Principles of Balance and Harmony 3

    The Benefits of Ayurveda 5

    Modern Relevance 8

Chapter 2: The Three Doshas 13

    Understanding Doshas: Vata, Pitta, and Kapha Explained 13

    Dosha Quiz: How to Determine Your Primary Dosha ... 16

    Balancing Doshas: The Importance of Maintaining Dosha Balance 20

Chapter 3: Ayurvedic Diet and Nutrition 23

    Foods for Each Dosha 26

    Seasonal Eating: Adjusting Your Diet With The Seasons 29

    The Art of Meal Planning & General Tips 32

Chapter 4: Daily Routines (Dinacharya) 35

The Importance of Routine 36

Morning Rituals: Starting the Day Right with
Ayurvedic Practices 38

Evening Rituals: Wind-Down Techniques for
Better Sleep 42

Personalizing Your Routine: Adapting Routines to Your
Lifestyle and Dosha 45

Chapter 5: Ayurvedic Detoxification (Panchakarma) 49

Types of Panchakarma 52

Home Detox Techniques: Simple Practices
for Beginners 55

When to Seek Professional Help: Understanding
Your Limits 57

Chapter 6: Ayurvedic Herbs and Supplements 61

Common Ayurvedic Herbs 64

Neem 79

Making Herbal Preparations: Teas, Tinctures,
and Powders 85

Safety and Dosage: Guidelines for Using Herbs
Responsibly 89

Chapter 7: Ayurvedic Bodywork and Self-Care 91

Abhyanga (Self-Massage) 92

Shirodhara: Oil Pouring Therapy for Stress Relief 94

Table of Contents

Marma Therapy: The Art of Energy Point Massage......97

Integrating Self-Care Practices 100

Chapter 8: Mind-Body Connection 103

Meditation and Mindfulness: Techniques
For Calming the Mind 106

Pranayama: Breathing Techniques for Energy
and Balance..108

Managing Stress and Emotions: Ayurvedic
Approaches to Mental Well-being................................... 110

Chapter 9: An Ayurvedic Approach to Exercise 115

Exercise and Doshas: Finding the Right Type
of Exercise for Your Dosha 116

Yoga and Ayurveda: The Synergy Between
Yoga and Ayurvedic Practices.. 118

Creating an Exercise Routine: Tips for a
Balanced and Sustainable Practice 121

Recovery and Rest: Importance of Rest
in Maintaining Health 122

Chapter 10: Ayurveda and Disease Prevention 127

Strengthening Immunity: Ayurvedic Practices
for a Robust Immune System 130

Understanding Disease in Ayurveda: Causes and
Progression of Diseases...134

Common Ailments and Remedies: Ayurvedic
Solutions for Everyday Issues. 137

Chapter 11: Ayurveda Across the Lifespan 141

    Ayurvedic Practices for Different Life Stages: Childhood, Adulthood, and Old Age 141

    Pregnancy and Postpartum Care: Special Considerations for Mothers 145

    Aging Gracefully: Ayurvedic Strategies for Healthy Aging 147

    Adapting Practices Over Time: How to Evolve Your Routine With Age 151

Chapter 12: Integrating Ayurveda into Modern Life 155

    Challenges and Solutions: Common Obstacles in Adopting Ayurveda and How to Overcome Them 155

    Combining Ayurveda with Other Health Practices: Finding a Balance with Modern Medicine 158

    Community and Resources: Finding Support and Further Learning 161

    Personal Stories and Testimonials 166

Conclusion 169

References 173

About the Author 177

Chapter 1

Introduction to Ayurveda

Welcome to the wonderful, spiritual, and fascinating world of Ayurveda. Right now, you might not know too much about this ancient practice, but by the end of this book, you'll know enough to embark on your own journey.

So, to help you get started, let's roll back to the beginning.

Ayurveda, often referred to as the "Science of Life," is a holistic system of medicine that originated in ancient India over 5000 years ago. The word Ayurveda comes from the Sanskrit words "ayur," meaning life, and "veda" meaning knowledge, emphasizing the interconnectedness of body, mind, and spirit in the maintenance of health and well-being.

The origins of Ayurveda can be traced back to the Vedas, the ancient scriptures of India, where the principles of Ayurveda were first documented. The fundamental texts of Ayurveda, known as the Charaka Samhita and the Sushruta Samhita, were compiled around 1000 BC and are considered the foundational texts of Ayurvedic medicine.

At its core, Ayurveda recognizes the importance of maintaining balance to achieve optimal health and prevent disease. Imbalances are believed to be the root cause of illness and disease, and Ayurvedic treatments aim to restore this balance through a combination of dietary modifications, herbal remedies, lifestyle changes, and therapeutic practices.

In addition to its focus on the individual, Ayurveda also places a strong emphasis on prevention, promoting healthy lifestyle practices such as daily routines, seasonal detoxification, and mindfulness practices to maintain overall well-being.

Over the centuries, Ayurveda has evolved and adapted to different cultures and regions, gaining recognition as a comprehensive system of medicine that encompasses not only physical health but also mental, emotional, and spiritual well-being. Today, Ayurveda is practiced worldwide, offering a unique perspective on health and healing that continues to inspire and influence the field of holistic medicine.

As we delve deeper into the world of Ayurveda, we'll uncover a treasure trove of wisdom that has withstood the test of time, offering a holistic approach to health and wellness that is as relevant and effective today as it was thousands of years ago. The principles of Ayurveda remind us of the interconnectedness of all aspects of our being and the importance of nurturing harmony within ourselves and our environment.

Philosophical Foundations: The Core Principles of Balance and Harmony

Picture this: Imagine a serene garden filled with vibrant flowers swaying gently in the breeze. In this peaceful setting, the principles of Ayurveda come to life, rooted in the idea that true health and well-being stem from a harmonious balance of mind, body, and spirit.

At the heart of Ayurveda lies the concept of the three doshas – Vata, Pitta, and Kapha. These doshas represent the fundamental energies that govern all biological functions within the body. Just like the elements of nature – air, fire, water, earth, and ether – each dosha carries its own unique qualities and characteristics.

Vata, embodying the elements of air and ether, governs movement and communication in the body. It is associated with qualities such as creativity, flexibility, and enthusiasm. Pitta, aligned with the elements of fire and water, governs transformation and metabolism. It is characterized by qualities like intensity, focus, and determination. Kapha, representing the elements of earth and water, governs structure and stability. It exudes qualities of nurturing, strength, and resilience.

In Ayurveda, the key to maintaining health and well-being lies in keeping these doshas in a state of balance. When any one of the doshas becomes excessive or deficient, it can lead to imbalances and, ultimately, disease. By understanding our unique constitution, or "prakriti," we can tailor our lifestyle, diet, and daily routines to support our individual needs and promote optimal health.

It's a little like your body as a finely tuned instrument, with each dosha playing its own melody in perfect harmony. When all three doshas are in balance, you experience a sense of vitality, clarity, and inner peace. It's like finding the perfect rhythm in a symphony of life, where every note blends seamlessly into the next.

Ayurveda teaches us to listen to our body's subtle cues and to be attuned to the ebb and flow of our inner landscape. Just as the seasons change, so too do the dynamics of our doshas. By adapting our lifestyle and habits according to these natural rhythms, we can align ourselves with the cyclical nature of existence.

In the quest for balance and harmony, Ayurveda offers a treasure trove of holistic practices, from herbal remedies and dietary recommendations to yoga, meditation, and pranayama (breathwork). Each of these modalities serves as a tool for cultivating self-awareness and fostering inner equilibrium.

As you explore the philosophical foundations of Ayurveda, you begin to see your body not as a separate entity but as an integral part of the intricate web of life. You realize that true health is not merely the absence of disease but a state of vibrant well-being that emanates from a deep sense of balance and wholeness.

By embracing the core principles of balance and harmony in Ayurveda, you embark on a transformative journey of self-care and self-discovery. You learn to cultivate a deeper connection with your body, mind, and spirit, nurturing a sense of wholeness that transcends the boundaries of individuality.

The Benefits of Ayurveda

Now that we know what Ayurveda is, let's talk about its incredible benefits and how it promotes health and well-being.

Personalized Approach:

- Ayurveda recognizes that each individual is unique and has a specific mind-body constitution known as doshas (Vata, Pitta, and Kapha).

- By identifying your dosha through a consultation with an Ayurvedic practitioner, you can tailor your diet, lifestyle, and wellness routines to suit your specific needs.

Emphasis on Prevention:

- Ayurveda focuses on preventing disease by maintaining balance in the body through practices such as yoga, meditation, and herbal remedies.
- By understanding your dosha and following Ayurvedic lifestyle guidelines, you can proactively prevent imbalances and health issues.

Natural Healing:

- Ayurveda utilizes natural remedies derived from herbs, minerals, and plants to address health concerns.
- These natural remedies are gentle on the body and promote healing without the harmful side effects often associated with synthetic medications.

Mind-Body Connection:

- Ayurveda recognizes the interconnectedness of the mind, body, and spirit in maintaining overall health.
- Practices such as meditation and pranayama (breathwork) are used to calm the mind, reduce stress, and promote emotional well-being.

Holistic Wellness:

- Ayurveda considers all aspects of your life, including diet, exercise, sleep, and mental health, in promoting holistic well-being.
- By addressing imbalances in all areas of life, Ayurveda aims to create harmony and vitality in the body.

Improved Digestion:

- Ayurveda places great emphasis on the importance of digestion in overall health.
- By following a diet tailored to your dosha and incorporating digestive spices and herbs, you can improve digestion and nutrient absorption.

Detoxification:

- Ayurveda promotes the practice of seasonal detoxification to eliminate toxins accumulated in the body.
- Through practices such as Panchakarma, a detox program involving therapies like massage and herbal cleanses, you can reset your body and promote optimal health.

Enhanced Energy Levels:

- By aligning with your natural doshic balance and incorporating Ayurvedic practices into your daily routine, you can experience increased energy levels and vitality.

- Ayurveda helps to remove blockages in the body's energy channels, known as nadis, allowing for improved energy flow.

Stress Reduction:

- Ayurveda offers various techniques, such as meditation, yoga, and stress-relieving herbal remedies, to help you manage and reduce stress.

- By addressing the root causes of stress and promoting relaxation, Ayurveda aids in maintaining mental clarity and emotional balance.

As you can see, Ayurveda is a comprehensive system of healing that offers a wealth of benefits for promoting health and well-being. From personalized approaches to natural remedies, Ayurveda provides you with the tools to achieve balance in mind, body, and spirit.

Modern Relevance

Let's explore how Ayurveda's ancient wisdom continues to be relevant in our modern world! Ayurveda, with its holistic approach to health and well-being, has stood the test of time and continues to be a valuable resource in contemporary health practices. Here's how Ayurveda fits seamlessly into our modern lifestyles:

- **Mind-Body Connection:** In today's fast-paced world, the importance of the mind-body connection is increasingly recognized in mainstream healthcare. Ayurveda's emphasis on the interconnectedness of physical health, mental well-being, and emotional balance aligns perfectly with modern approaches to holistic health.

- **Personalized Medicine:** The rise of personalized medicine and integrative healthcare has brought Ayurveda to the forefront as a valuable tool for understanding individual health needs. Ayurvedic principles of doshas help individuals customize their diet, lifestyle, and wellness routines to optimize their health outcomes.

- **Natural Remedies:** With our growing interest in natural and holistic healing modalities, Ayurveda's reliance on natural remedies derived from herbs, minerals, and plants resonates with modern consumers seeking non-invasive health solutions. Ayurvedic herbs and supplements are increasingly gaining popularity for their effectiveness and minimal side effects compared to synthetic medications.

- **Preventive Healthcare:** As the focus shifts towards preventive healthcare and wellness promotion, Ayurveda's emphasis on maintaining balance in the body to prevent disease is particularly relevant. Ayurvedic practices such as yoga, meditation, and seasonal detoxification offer practical tools to take charge of our health and well-being proactively.

- **Stress Management:** We all know how stressful modern society has become, and because of that, stress management has become a crucial aspect of overall health. Ayurveda's holistic approach to stress reduction through practices like meditation, pranayama, and herbal remedies provides effective tools for us to combat stress and promote mental resilience.

- **Digestive Health:** With digestive issues on the rise due to poor diet and lifestyle choices, Ayurveda's focus on improving digestion through dietary recommendations tailored to one's dosha is highly relevant. Ayurvedic principles of mindful eating and digestion-enhancing spices offer practical solutions for improving gut health and nutrient absorption.

- **Integrative Wellness:** Ayurveda seamlessly integrates with other wellness practices such as yoga, acupuncture, and mindfulness meditation to create a comprehensive approach to health and well-being. By incorporating Ayurvedic principles into a holistic wellness routine, you can enhance the effectiveness of other modalities and achieve optimal health outcomes.

- **Eco-Friendly Living:** As sustainability and eco-consciousness become key considerations in modern lifestyles, Ayurveda's emphasis on living in harmony with nature aligns perfectly with the ethos of environmental conservation. Ayurvedic practices encourage eco-friendly habits such as eating seasonally, using natural and organic products, and minimizing waste to promote a healthier planet and a healthier self.

By embracing Ayurveda's principles and incorporating them into our daily lives, we can tap into the ancient wisdom that continues to guide us towards a more balanced, vibrant, and healthy existence.

Chapter 2

The Three Doshas

We've already touched upon the idea of doshas. But you need to know more, right? In this chapter, we delve further into the fundamental building blocks of Ayurvedic philosophy.

According to Ayurveda, each person is made up of a unique combination of three Doshas - Vata, Pitta, and Kapha - which govern our physical, mental, and emotional characteristics. Understanding your dominant Dosha can offer deep insights into your natural tendencies, strengths, and potential imbalances.

Let's jump in!

Understanding Doshas: Vata, Pitta, and Kapha Explained

To appreciate the power of doshas, you need to learn about each one in turn. Let's do that now.

Vata, the Air and Space Energy

Picture a whimsical dancer moving gracefully through the wind. That's Vata, the dosha associated with the elements of air and space. Vata governs movement, creativity, and communication in our bodies and minds. If you have a Vata constitution, you might be quick-witted, adaptable, and bursting with ideas. Your energy is like the wind - unpredictable, changing, and always in motion.

However, when Vata is out of balance, you may experience anxiety, restlessness, and scattered thoughts. It's crucial for Vata types to find grounding practices like meditation, yoga, or regular routines to calm the whirlwind of the mind. Nourishing, warm foods and self-care rituals can also help balance Vata energy and bring stability to your life.

Pitta, the Fire Energy

Now, let's turn up the heat and meet Pitta, the fiery dosha driven by the elements of fire and water. Pitta governs digestion, metabolism, and transformation in our bodies and minds. If you are a Pitta type, you are likely a natural leader with a sharp intellect, strong drive, and a fiery passion for life. Your energy is like a blazing fire - intense, focused, and full of ambition.

But when Pitta is imbalanced, you may experience irritability, perfectionism, and burnout. Cooling practices like swimming, spending time in nature, or enjoying cooling foods can help soothe Pitta's intense flames. Learning to let go of control, practicing relaxation techniques, and maintaining a balanced diet are key to keeping Pitta's energy in check and maintaining harmony within yourself.

Kapha, the Earth, and Water Energy

Lastly, let's take a deep breath and sink into the nurturing embrace of Kapha, the dosha ruled by the elements of earth and water. Kapha governs structure, stability, and endurance in our bodies and minds. If you have a Kapha constitution, you are likely calm, compassionate, and grounded, with a strong sense of loyalty and love for routine. Your energy is like a gentle stream - steady, nurturing, and deeply rooted.

However, when Kapha is out of balance, you may experience lethargy, attachment, and resistance to change. Engaging in stimulating activities, incorporating movement into your daily routine, and enjoying warming spices can help invigorate Kapha energy and bring vitality back into your life. Finding ways to challenge yourself, practicing gratitude, and embracing new experiences are essential for Kapha types to maintain balance and harmony.

Remember, we all have a unique combination of Vata, Pitta, and Kapha energies within us, and achieving balance is a lifelong journey. By understanding the qualities of each dosha and recognizing their effects on your body and mind, you can make informed choices to support your well-being and lead a harmonious life.

Dosha Quiz: How to Determine Your Primary Dosha

Your next question is sure to be about your own primary dosha. Well, look no further! This quiz will help you unravel the mysteries of your primary dosha, Vata, Pitta, or Kapha.

1. What best describes your body frame?

a) Thin, wiry, or slender

b) Medium build, athletic, or muscular

c) Solid, sturdy, or curvy

2. How do you usually respond to stress?

a) I tend to feel anxious, restless, and overwhelmed.

b) I become irritable, impatient, and demanding.

c) I feel lethargic, unmotivated, and withdrawn.

3. What is your skin type?

a) Dry, rough, or may experience skin conditions like eczema

b) Sensitive, prone to redness or inflammation, may have acne

c) Smooth, oily, or well-hydrated

4. When it comes to food, what do you crave the most?

a) Light and crunchy snacks like popcorn or crackers

b) Spicy and tangy flavors like salsa or jalapenos

c) Comforting and heavy meals like pasta or mashed potatoes

5. Which climate do you prefer?

a) Warm and humid weather

b) Hot and dry climate

c) Cool and damp environment

6. How do you handle tasks and projects?

a) I am creative and imaginative, but I may struggle with follow-through.

b) I am organized, driven, and goal-oriented.

c) I am methodical, patient, and prefer routine

7. What is your sleep pattern like?

a) I have difficulty falling asleep and often wake up during the night.

b) I have intense dreams and may wake up feeling hot.

c) I am a deep sleeper and sometimes struggle to wake up in the morning.

8. How do you communicate with others?

a) I am articulate but may ramble or lose track of the conversation.

b) I am assertive, direct, and sometimes critical.

c) I am a good listener and tend to speak slowly and thoughtfully.

9. What physical issues do you experience most frequently?

a) Digestive issues like gas, bloating, or constipation

b) Inflammation, acid reflux, or skin irritations

c) Slow metabolism, weight gain, or sinus congestion

10. How do you unwind and relax?

a) Engaging in creative activities like painting or writing

b) Exercising or doing intense physical activities

c) Taking hot baths, meditating, or spending time in nature

Now, let's discover your dominant dosha based on your responses.

If you answered mostly a's:

Congratulations! You are predominantly Vata! Your mind-body type is characterized by creativity, enthusiasm, and sensitivity. Embrace practices that ground and nurture your Vata nature, such as warm meals, calming activities, and routines.

If you answered mostly b's:

You are predominantly Pitta! Your dosha embodies passion, focus, and intensity. Balance your Pitta tendencies with cooling practices, relaxation techniques, and mindfulness to maintain harmony in body and mind.

If you answered mostly c's:

You are predominantly Kapha! Your dosha exudes stability, compassion, and endurance. Embrace invigorating activities, light foods, and movement to keep your Kapha energy balanced and vibrant.

Remember, Ayurveda is all about finding balance and harmony within yourself. Your dosha may change over time or vary depending on the seasons and circumstances.

Balancing Doshas: The Importance of Maintaining Dosha Balance

We know that the doshas are the three vital energies that govern our physical and mental well-being. These doshas - Vata, Pitta, and Kapha - are derived from the five elements: ether, air, fire, water, and earth. Each dosha has its own unique qualities and functions in our body. Balancing these doshas is key to maintaining good health, vitality, and harmony within ourselves.

Let's start with Vata dosha, which is associated with movement and is composed of ether and air elements. Vata governs all bodily functions related to movement, such as breathing, circulation, and nerve impulses. When Vata is in balance, it promotes creativity, agility, and enthusiasm. However, when Vata is aggravated, it can lead to anxiety, insomnia, and digestive issues. To balance Vata, it's important to follow a routine, stay warm, practice grounding exercises like yoga, and eat warm, nourishing foods.

Next up is Pitta dosha, which is related to metabolism and transformation and is made up of fire and water elements. Pitta controls digestion, metabolism, and hormones. When Pitta is balanced, it enhances intelligence, courage, and passion. On the flip side, an excess of Pitta can manifest as irritability, inflammation, and skin issues. To keep Pitta in check, it's recommended to stay cool, practice relaxation techniques, eat cooling foods, and avoid spicy and greasy foods.

Last but not least, we have Kapha dosha, which embodies structure and stability and is a combination of earth and water elements. Kapha regulates strength, immunity, and lubrication in the body. When Kapha is balanced, it promotes love, compassion, and stability. Yet, when Kapha becomes imbalanced, it can lead to lethargy, weight gain, and respiratory issues. To maintain Kapha equilibrium, it's beneficial to stay active, incorporate stimulating activities, eat light and spicy foods, and avoid heavy, sweet, and dairy-laden meals.

Once you identify your dosha type, you can tailor your lifestyle, diet, and activities to harmonize your doshas.

To maintain dosha balance, Ayurveda emphasizes the importance of following a daily routine, or dinacharya. This routine includes practices like waking up early, scraping the tongue, oil pulling, self-massage with warm oil, and meditation. Establishing a consistent routine helps regulate your biological clock, promotes digestion, and calms the mind.

In addition to a daily routine, diet plays a crucial role in balancing doshas. Ayurveda categorizes foods based on their taste (rasa), energy (virya), and post-digestive effect (vipaka) to determine their effects on doshas. For instance, sweet, sour, and salty tastes pacify Vata, while bitter, astringent, and pungent tastes pacify Kapha.

When it comes to lifestyle habits, incorporating regular exercise, adequate sleep, stress management techniques, and self-care practices are essential for dosha balance. Engage in activities that bring joy and relaxation, such as nature walks, aromatherapy, yoga, or spending time with loved ones.

Remember, listening to your body and being mindful of how you feel physically, emotionally, and mentally is key to maintaining dosha equilibrium. If you notice any signs of dosha imbalance, such as digestive issues, skin problems, mood swings, or fatigue, listen to your body's signals and make the necessary adjustments to restore balance.

Chapter 3

Ayurvedic Diet and Nutrition

Ayurveda has long emphasized the significance of food in maintaining health and promoting overall well-being. According to Ayurvedic principles, food is not just nourishment for the body but also a form of medicine that can prevent diseases, balance energies within the body, and promote longevity.

To help you learn more, let's delve into the fascinating world of Ayurvedic dietary principles and explore how the choices we make in our daily meals can have a profound impact on our health.

In Ayurveda, food is classified based on its taste (rasa), its effect on the body post-digestion (vipaka), and its heating or cooling properties (virya). These classifications help determine the inherent qualities of different foods and how they interact with the body's doshas (basic physiological energies): – Vata, Pitta, and Kapha.

Vata, associated with the elements of air and ether, is characterized by qualities such as being cold, light, dry, and mobile. Pitta, governed by the elements of fire and water, is characterized by qualities such as being hot, sharp, and intense. Kapha, associated with the elements of earth and water, is characterized by qualities such as being heavy, slow, and stable. If this makes little sense right now, don't worry! We're going to talk about food for each dosha in the next section.

In Ayurveda, the concept of Agni (digestive fire) is very important. A strong Agni is essential for proper digestion, assimilation of nutrients, and elimination of waste products. To nourish Agni, it is advised to eat mindfully, chew food thoroughly, and avoid overeating or consuming incompatible food combinations.

Ayurveda also emphasizes the importance of eating according to the seasons and your constitution. For example, during the cold winter months, it is beneficial to favor warm, cooked foods that are grounding and nourishing. On the other hand, during the hot summer months, opting for light, cooling foods can help balance Pitta and prevent overheating.

Continuing with the same idea, Ayurveda considers food not just in terms of its physical properties but also its prana (life force) and its effect on the mind and emotions. Consuming fresh, organic, and locally sourced foods is believed to be more energetically vibrant and supportive of overall health.

One of the key principles of Ayurvedic dietary guidelines is the practice of Sattvic eating, which focuses on pure, wholesome foods that promote clarity, vitality, and balance. Sattvic foods include fresh fruits and vegetables, whole grains, nuts, seeds, and dairy products in moderation. By consuming Sattvic foods, you can cultivate a sense of inner peace and harmony.

Ayurveda also recognizes the concept of food as medicine (Bhavaprakash Nighantu), wherein specific foods are prescribed to treat various imbalances or diseases. For example, turmeric is revered for its anti-inflammatory properties, ginger is used to aid digestion, and ghee is considered a nourishing tonic for the body.

In addition to choosing the right foods, Ayurveda also emphasizes the importance of mindful eating practices. This includes eating in a calm and peaceful environment, free from distractions, savoring each bite, and expressing gratitude for the nourishment provided by the food.

There is also the concept of Aharvidhi Vidhan to consider, which involves guidelines for how to eat to promote optimal digestion and assimilation of nutrients. This includes eating only when hungry, avoiding excessive snacking between meals, and allowing for proper time gaps between meals for digestion to occur efficiently.

Ayurveda also recognizes the individuality of each person and the need for personalized dietary recommendations based on one's unique constitution (Prakriti) and imbalances (Vikriti). By understanding one's doshic makeup and current state of health, you can make informed choices about the foods that will best support your well-being.

As you can see, it's about doing what is right for you and your specific dosha. So, let's talk about the foods you should eat and avoid depending on your main dosha type.

Foods for Each Dosha

We touched upon what types of foods each dosha "likes," but what does that look like in practice? What should you eat versus what you should avoid? Let's learn more.

Vata Dosha

Vata, associated with the elements of air and ether, is characterized by qualities such as being cold, light, dry, and mobile.

What to Eat:

- Warm, nourishing, and grounding foods such as cooked grains, root vegetables, warm soups, stews, and herbal teas.

- Dairy products like warm milk and ghee are beneficial for balancing Vata.
- Sweet, sour, and salty tastes help pacify Vata dosha.
- Nuts, seeds, and oils provide essential fats for the Vata constitution.

What to Avoid:

- Cold, dry, and raw foods can aggravate Vata dosha.
- Bitter, astringent, and pungent tastes should be consumed in moderation.
- Caffeinated beverages and excessive intake of sugar can disturb Vata balance.
- Avoid processed foods and carbonated drinks.

Pitta Dosha

Pitta, governed by the elements of fire and water, is characterized by qualities such as being hot, sharp, and intense.

What to Eat:

- Cooling, and hydrating foods such as cucumber, mint, coconut, and coriander are beneficial for Pitta dosha.
- Sweet, bitter, and astringent tastes help balance the fiery nature of Pitta.

- Vegetables like broccoli, cauliflower, and leafy greens are great choices for Pitta individuals.
- Moderate amounts of grains, legumes, and cooling spices like fennel and coriander can help pacify Pitta dosha.

What to Avoid:

- Spicy, oily, and fried foods can exacerbate Pitta dosha.
- Sour and salty tastes should be consumed in moderation.
- Avoid excessive intake of caffeine and alcohol.
- Limit consumption of red meat and processed foods.

Kapha Dosha

Kapha, associated with the elements of earth and water, is characterized by qualities such as heavy, slow, and stable.

What to Eat:

- Light, dry, and warm foods help balance Kapha dosha. Incorporate plenty of cooked vegetables, grains, and legumes into your diet.
- Pungent, bitter, and astringent tastes help reduce Kapha's heaviness.
- Spices like ginger, black pepper, and turmeric can aid digestion and metabolism in Kapha individuals.

- Fruits like apples, pears, and berries are suitable choices for the Kapha constitution.

What to Avoid:

- Heavy, oily, and sweet foods can worsen Kapha imbalance.
- Dairy products and excess consumption of nuts should be limited.
- Avoid cold and excessively moist foods.
- Minimize your intake of sugary and processed foods.

Remember, Ayurveda emphasizes the importance of listening to your body's unique needs and adjusting your diet accordingly. Experiment with different foods and observe how your body responds to find the optimal balance for your dosha type.

Seasonal Eating: Adjusting Your Diet With The Seasons

According to Ayurveda, each season brings with it a unique energy that influences our bodies, minds, and overall well-being. By aligning our diets with the rhythms of nature, we can tap into the healing power of seasonal foods and support our body's innate ability to thrive.

Let's dive into the magic of seasonal eating through an Ayurvedic lens:

Embracing the Wisdom of Nature

In Ayurveda, it is believed that nature provides us with everything we need to nourish and heal ourselves. By eating foods that are in season, we can harness the vital energies present in fresh, locally sourced produce. In the spring, opt for lighter, cleansing foods like leafy greens, sprouts, and berries to support detoxification and renewal.

As summer rolls around, indulge in juicy fruits, cooling vegetables, and hydrating foods to balance the heat and Pitta dosha. Come fall, embrace hearty root vegetables, warming spices, and nourishing soups to ground Vata energy, and prepare for the winter ahead.

Balancing the Doshas

Ayurveda recognizes three primary doshas – Vata, Pitta, and Kapha – that govern our physical, mental, and emotional well-being. Each season is associated with a different dosha, and adjusting your diet to pacify the dominant dosha can help maintain equilibrium within the body. For example, during the cold, dry Vata season of fall and early winter, opt for foods that are grounding, nourishing, and warming to counterbalance Vata's erratic qualities.

In the fiery Pitta season of summer, focus on cooling, hydrating foods to soothe Pitta's intensity. In the wet, heavy Kapha season of spring, choose light, spicy foods to stimulate digestion and uplift Kapha energy.

Connecting with the Elemental Energies

Ayurveda views the world through the lens of the five elements – earth, water, fire, air, and ether – and believes that these elements influence all aspects of our being, including our dietary needs. Each season is associated with a unique combination of these elements, and by tuning into the elemental energies of nature, we can choose foods that resonate with the current season. For example, the earthy and grounding qualities of root vegetables like sweet potatoes and carrots are perfect for fall, while the fiery and transformative nature of spices like ginger and turmeric is ideal for winter.

By embracing these elemental energies, we can attune ourselves to the natural rhythms of the universe and find greater balance within.

Cultivating Mindful Eating

Seasonal eating is not just about nourishing the body; it is also a practice of mindfulness and gratitude. By savoring the flavors, textures, and aromas of seasonal foods, we can deepen our connection to the earth and the abundance it provides. Take the time to appreciate the vibrant colors of a ripe summer tomato, the earthy sweetness of a winter squash, or the crisp freshness of a spring salad.

Engage all your senses in the act of eating, and allow yourself to be fully present with each bite. In doing so, you not only nourish your body but also feed your soul.

Experimenting with Seasonal Recipes

One of the joys of seasonal eating is the opportunity to get creative in the kitchen and experiment with new flavors and combinations. Try incorporating seasonal ingredients into your favorite recipes or exploring traditional Ayurvedic dishes tailored to the current season. Whip up a batch of hearty lentil soup with winter root vegetables, infuse your summer salads with cooling mint and cilantro, or indulge in a nourishing stew of spring greens and spices.

Let your imagination run wild and allow the seasonal bounty to inspire your culinary creations.

The Art of Meal Planning & General Tips

Meal planning in Ayurveda is not just about what you eat, but also when and how you eat it. By understanding your dosha and incorporating Ayurvedic principles into your meal planning, you can optimize your health and well-being.

Here are some tips to help you get started:

- **Include All Six Tastes:** Ayurveda recognizes six tastes: sweet, sour, salty, bitter, pungent, and astringent. A balanced meal should include all six tastes in order to satisfy your palate and nourish your body. For example, a meal could consist of grains (sweet), lemon (sour), salted vegetables (salty), leafy greens (bitter), ginger (pungent), and beans (astringent).

- **Mindful Eating:** Ayurveda emphasizes the importance of being present while eating. Take the time to sit down and savor your meals without distractions. Chew your food thoroughly to aid digestion and appreciate the flavors and textures of each bite.

- **Create a Routine:** Establishing a regular meal schedule can help regulate your digestion and metabolism. Aim to eat your meals at the same time each day to support your body's natural rhythms.

- **Cook with Love:** In Ayurveda, the energy and intention you put into cooking can impact the quality of your food. When preparing meals, infuse them with love and positive energy to enhance their nourishing effects on your body and mind.

- **Herbs and Spices:** Incorporating Ayurvedic herbs and spices into your cooking can enhance the healing properties of your meals. Turmeric, ginger, cumin, and coriander are just a few examples of spices known for their medicinal benefits.

- **Listen to Your Body:** Pay attention to how your body responds to different foods. Notice any digestive issues, energy levels, or mood changes after eating certain meals. Adjust your diet accordingly to maintain balance and well-being.

- **Plan Ahead:** Taking the time to plan your meals in advance can save you time and stress during the week. Make a shopping list, prep ingredients, and cook in batches to have healthy meals ready when you need them.

- **Stay Hydrated:** Drinking plenty of water throughout the day is essential for proper digestion and detoxification. In Ayurveda, warm water is often recommended to help eliminate toxins and balance the doshas.

By incorporating these Ayurvedic principles into your meal planning, you can create a nourishing and balanced diet that supports your overall health and well-being.

Chapter 4

Daily Routines (Dinacharya)

Dinacharya, a key concept in Ayurveda, refers to daily routines and practices that are believed to promote health and well-being by aligning the body with the natural daily rhythms of the universe. The word "Dinacharya" is derived from Sanskrit, with "Dina" meaning day and "Charya" meaning conduct or care.

In Ayurveda, it is believed that following a consistent dinacharya helps to maintain balance in the body and mind, preventing disease and promoting longevity. The dinacharya practices are tailored to your constitution or dosha.

A typical dinacharya includes practices such as waking up early in the morning before sunrise, practicing gentle yoga or stretching, cleansing the body through practices like tongue scraping and oil pulling, and engaging in meditation or mindfulness exercises. Other important aspects of dinacharya include regular meal times, specific dietary guidelines, and maintaining a bedtime routine to ensure adequate rest and rejuvenation.

Let's delve more into why routine is so important in Ayurveda and how you can create your own.

The Importance of Routine

Imagine a world where your daily habits not only impact your physical health but also influence your mental, emotional, and spiritual well-being. This is the philosophy that Ayurveda is built upon. Ayurveda teaches us that our habits can either nourish or deplete our life force, known as "prana," and that establishing a healthy daily routine is key to achieving balance and harmony within our bodies and minds.

In Ayurveda, the concept of "dinacharya," or daily routine, is emphasized as a fundamental aspect of health maintenance. By following a consistent routine that aligns with your unique mind-body type, or dosha, you can enhance your overall well-being and reduce the risk of imbalances and illness.

One of the core principles of Ayurveda is that each of us is unique, with our own specific constitution and needs. This is why it's essential to tailor your daily routine to suit your own doshic balance. For example, a person with a predominance of the Vata dosha may benefit from grounding practices, such as a warm oil massage before bathing, while someone with a Pitta constitution may thrive on cooling activities like taking a leisurely walk by the water.

One of the key ways in which routine impacts health in Ayurveda is through the concept of "agni," or digestive fire. According to Ayurvedic philosophy, a strong and balanced agni is essential for proper digestion, absorption, and assimilation of nutrients. By establishing healthy eating habits, such as eating regular meals at consistent times, avoiding heavy or processed foods, and taking time to savor and appreciate each bite, you can support your agni and promote optimal digestion.

In addition to diet, Ayurveda places great importance on daily practices that support overall well-being, such as proper sleep, exercise, and stress management. Establishing a regular sleep schedule, engaging in physical activity that aligns with your dosha, and incorporating mindfulness practices like meditation or pranayama can all contribute to a healthier and more balanced life.

Additionally, the mind-body connection is at the heart of Ayurveda, with the understanding that our thoughts, emotions, and beliefs can have a profound impact on our physical health. Incorporating practices that nourish the mind, such as journaling, gratitude exercises, or spending time in nature, can help to cultivate a positive mindset and promote emotional well-being.

By embracing the wisdom of Ayurveda and incorporating its principles into your daily routine, you can create a lifestyle that not only supports your physical health but also nurtures your mind and spirit. Remember, consistency is key when it comes to establishing new habits, so start small and gradually build upon your routine to create a personalized practice that resonates with you.

It's time to embrace the power of routine, prioritize self-care, and watch as your overall well-being blossoms like a beautifully tended garden. Your future self will thank you for it!

Morning Rituals: Starting the Day Right with Ayurvedic Practices

Let's start with the moment you open your eyes. By incorporating Ayurvedic practices into your morning routine, you can set the tone for a day filled with intention, energy, and well-being.

Wake Up with the Sun

In Ayurveda, the hours before sunrise are known as the "Brahma Muhurta," a time of day that is considered most conducive to spiritual practices and mental clarity. By aligning your waking time with the rising sun, you not only synchronize your body's internal clock but also tap into the potent energy of a new day.

As the first rays of sunlight gently kiss your eyelids, take a moment to express gratitude for the gift of another day. Welcome the day with a gentle smile and a heart full of appreciation for the opportunities and experiences that lie ahead.

Practice Abhyanga: Self-Massage with Warm Oil

One of the foundational practices in Ayurveda is Abhyanga, the art of self-massage using warm oil. This nourishing ritual helps to nourish the skin, soothe the nervous system, and promote lymphatic flow. Before stepping into the shower, take a few minutes to massage your body with warm sesame or coconut oil, moving in gentle, circular motions towards the heart.

As you massage your skin, offer loving kindness to yourself, and honor the sacred temple that houses your spirit. Feel the warmth of the oil seep into your pores, bringing a sense of grounding and tranquility to your being.

Cleanse Your Senses with Oil Pulling and Tongue Scraping

After your Abhyanga practice, indulge in the ancient Ayurvedic rituals of oil pulling and tongue scraping to cleanse your senses and promote oral hygiene. Oil pulling involves swishing a tablespoon of coconut or sesame oil in your mouth for 5–10 minutes, helping to remove toxins and bacteria from your oral cavity.

Following oil pulling, gently scrape your tongue with a copper or stainless steel tongue scraper to remove accumulated ama (toxins) and bacteria. This simple practice not only freshens your breath but also stimulates digestion and detoxification pathways in the body.

Hydrate Yourself with Warm Lemon Water

Before indulging in your breakfast, quench your body's thirst with a warm cup of lemon water. Squeeze half a fresh lemon into a cup of warm water and sip mindfully, relishing the invigorating tang of citrus and the soothing warmth of the liquid.

Lemon water not only hydrates the body after a night of fasting but also kickstarts your digestive fire (Agni) and alkalizes your system. Embrace this simple yet powerful ritual as a way to cleanse and rejuvenate your body from the inside out.

Practice Pranayama: Breathwork for Vitality

As you continue to awaken your body and mind, engage in the practice of Pranayama, or yogic breathwork, to cultivate inner vitality and mental clarity. Choose a simple breathing technique such as Nadi Shodhana (alternate nostril breathing) or Bhastrika (bellows breath) to invigorate your prana (life force) and balance your energy channels.

Sit comfortably in a quiet space, close your eyes, and place your hands on your belly. Inhale deeply through your nose, feeling your abdomen expand, then exhale fully, releasing any tension or stagnation from your being. Allow the rhythm of your breath to guide you into a state of presence and centeredness.

Set Intentions through Meditation and Visualization

Before stepping into the demands of the day, take a few moments to connect with your innermost desires and set clear intentions for how you wish to show up in the world. Find a comfortable seated position, close your eyes, and bring your awareness to your heart center.

Through the practice of meditation and visualization, invite feelings of abundance, joy, and purpose. Envision your day unfolding with grace and ease, affirming your worthiness and capability to handle whatever comes your way. Allow this sacred space of stillness to anchor you in the present moment and empower you to navigate the day with mindfulness and intention.

Nourish Your Body with a Sattvic Breakfast

As you conclude your morning rituals, honor your body's needs by nourishing it with a sattvic (pure) breakfast that supports your vitality and well-being. Choose whole, unprocessed foods such as fresh fruits, whole grains, nuts, and seeds to fuel your body with essential nutrients and prana.

Sit down mindfully to enjoy your breakfast, savoring each bite and expressing gratitude for the nourishment that sustains you. Cultivate a sense of reverence for the gifts of the earth and the interconnectedness of all beings as you receive the blessings of your morning meal.

Evening Rituals: Wind-Down Techniques for Better Sleep

As the sun begins to dip below the horizon and the hustle and bustle of the day gradually fade away, it's time to embrace the tranquility of the evening. Ayurveda places great emphasis on the importance of establishing rituals to support the natural rhythms of the body and mind. And truly, there's nothing quite like the feeling of sinking into bed, utterly at peace, and ready to drift off into dreamland.

To kick off your evening wind-down, let's start by setting the scene. Create a peaceful sanctuary in your bedroom by dimming the lights and lighting some soothing candles or incense. Play some gentle music or nature sounds to further enhance the relaxing ambiance.

Let's take a look at some Ayurvedic wind-down techniques to help you ease into a deep and restorative slumber.

Abhyanga (Self-Massage)

Treat yourself to a calming self-massage with warm, aromatic oils like sesame or coconut oil. In Ayurveda, this practice is known as Abhyanga and is believed to promote relaxation, improve circulation, and nourish the skin. As you massage your body in gentle, circular motions, take a few moments to appreciate and connect with your physical self.

Sip on Herbal Tea

Enjoy a cup of soothing herbal tea to help calm your mind and body. Ayurvedic favorites include chamomile, peppermint, or ashwagandha tea, which are known for their calming and relaxing properties. Sipping on a warm cup of tea can be a comforting way to wind down and signal to your body that it's time to relax.

Practice Pranayama

Engage in some gentle breathing exercises, such as Pranayama, to help calm the mind and release any tension or stress from the day. One popular Pranayama technique is Nadi Shodhana (alternate nostril breathing), which helps balance the energy channels in the body and promotes a sense of peace and relaxation.

Mindful Meditation

Take a few minutes to practice mindful meditation before bedtime. Sit comfortably, close your eyes, and focus on your breath as you let go of any racing thoughts or worries. Allow yourself to be fully present in the moment and acknowledge any sensations or emotions that arise without judgment. This practice can help quiet the mind and prepare you for a restful night's sleep.

Digital Detox

Unplug from electronic devices at least an hour before bedtime to reduce exposure to blue light, which can disrupt your natural sleep-wake cycle. Instead of scrolling through social media or watching TV, opt for activities that promote relaxation, such as reading a book, journaling, or simply enjoying some quiet time with yourself.

Warm Bath

Indulge in a warm bath infused with Epsom salts, lavender essential oil, or rose petals to help relax your muscles and soothe your senses. The combination of warm water and aromatherapy can be incredibly calming and rejuvenating, setting the stage for a blissful night of sleep.

Gratitude Practice

Before drifting off to sleep, take a moment to reflect on the day and express gratitude for the blessings and lessons it has brought. Cultivating a sense of gratitude can shift your focus from worries and stress to a sense of contentment and abundance, creating a positive mindset that can improve the quality of your sleep.

By incorporating these Ayurvedic wind-down techniques into your evening ritual, you can create a peaceful and nurturing bedtime routine that supports your overall well-being and helps you enjoy a restful night's sleep.

Personalizing Your Routine: Adapting Routines to Your Lifestyle and Dosha

Personalizing your routine involves understanding your dosha and adapting your lifestyle practices to bring balance and harmony to your mind, body, and spirit. By aligning your daily habits with your doshic makeup, you can optimize your overall well-being and enhance your natural vitality.

Now, the key to personalizing your routine lies in identifying your dominant dosha and making conscious choices that support its optimal expression. Here are some practical tips for adapting your daily habits to align with your doshic constitution:

Morning Routine

Start your day with a grounding ritual that resonates with your dosha. Vata types may benefit from gentle movements like yoga or tai chi to calm their active minds. Pitta individuals can embrace cooling practices such as meditation or breathing exercises to promote inner tranquility. Kapha personalities may find invigorating activities like brisk walks or dry brushing stimulating.

Dietary Choices

Tailor your diet to pacify your dominant dosha. Vata types can favor warm, nourishing foods like soups, stews, and cooked grains to soothe their delicate digestive systems. Pitta individuals should opt for cooling, hydrating foods such as salads, fresh fruits, and leafy greens to balance their fiery nature. Kapha personalities benefit from light, spicy dishes like stir-fries, lentil soups, and herbal teas to offset their tendency towards sluggishness.

Exercise Regimen

Select exercises that support your doshic constitution. Vata individuals thrive on activities that foster stability and focus, such as gentle yoga, swimming, or Pilates. Pitta types enjoy challenging workouts like running, cycling, or weight training to release excess energy. Kapha personalities find solace in dynamic practices like dance, aerobics, or martial arts to invigorate their sluggish metabolism.

Sleep Routine

Establish a bedtime routine that promotes restful sleep based on your dosha. Vata types benefit from calming activities like reading, journaling, or listening to calming music before bed to unwind their active minds. Pitta individuals should engage in relaxation techniques such as meditation, deep breathing, or progressive muscle relaxation to cool their fiery temperament. Kapha personalities can engage in stimulating practices like self-massage, dry brushing, or light stretching to counterbalance their tendency towards heaviness.

Self-Care Practices

Incorporate personalized self-care rituals into your daily routine to nurture your mind, body, and soul. Vata types may appreciate warm oil massages, aromatherapy, or grounding rituals to foster a sense of stability and comfort. Pitta individuals can benefit from cooling practices like rosewater mists, soothing baths, or mindful breathing exercises to soothe their sensitive nature. Kapha personalities find rejuvenation in invigorating activities like energetic yoga, dry brushing, or herbal steams to awaken their senses.

Remember, personalizing your routine is a journey of self-discovery and self-care. Embrace the uniqueness of your doshic constitution and honor your body's innate wisdom. By adapting your daily habits to support your dosha, you can cultivate balance, harmony, and vitality in all aspects of your life.

Chapter 5

Ayurvedic Detoxification (Panchakarma)

Panchakarma is an ancient Ayurvedic detoxification process that has been revered for centuries as a powerful method to cleanse not just the body but also the mind and spirit.

Panchakarma, derived from Sanskrit words meaning "five actions," is a comprehensive detoxification and rejuvenation protocol that is at the heart of Ayurvedic medicine. The primary goal of Panchakarma is to rid the body of accumulated toxins, or "ama," that are believed to be the root cause of disease and imbalance, according to Ayurvedic principles.

Imagine your body as a temple, a sacred vessel that needs regular maintenance and cleansing to function at its optimal level. In the same way, we declutter our living spaces, Panchakarma aims to declutter our physical and energetic bodies, allowing the natural healing mechanisms of the body to kick into high gear.

Detoxification in Ayurveda goes beyond the physical realm; it encompasses the mind, emotions, and spirit as well. Ayurveda recognizes that we are not just a collection of organs and tissues but a holistic being composed of interconnected layers of existence. The accumulation of toxins, or ama, can manifest as physical ailments, mental fog, emotional imbalances, and spiritual stagnation.

By undergoing Panchakarma or other detox protocols, we allow the body to release deep-seated toxins, rejuvenate cellular function, balance the doshas, and restore harmony to our being. Detoxification in Ayurveda is not about deprivation or harsh cleansing methods but about nurturing the body with healing foods, herbal remedies, self-care practices, and mindful living.

In addition to physical cleansing, detox in Ayurveda aims to reset the mind and emotions, creating space for clarity, peace, and joy to emerge. As toxins are released from the body, stagnant emotions, limiting beliefs, and mental clutter can also be purged, leading to a profound sense of lightness and clarity.

The Benefits of Panchakarma and Detox in Ayurveda

- **Rejuvenation and Vitality:** Panchakarma is like hitting the reset button for your entire being. By removing accumulated toxins and restoring balance to the doshas, you can experience renewed energy, vitality, and a sense of well-being.

- **Enhanced Digestion and Metabolism:** A clean digestive system is key to overall health, according to Ayurveda. Panchakarma helps improve digestive fire (agni), assimilation of nutrients, and elimination of waste, leading to improved metabolism and nutrient absorption.

- **Mental Clarity and Emotional Balance:** As the body detoxifies, the mind also experiences a cleansing process. Many individuals report feeling more mentally alert, emotionally stable, and spiritually connected after undergoing Panchakarma, or detoxification.

- **Stronger Immunity:** A healthy immune system is vital for warding off illnesses and maintaining optimal health. By eliminating toxins and restoring balance to the body, Panchakarma can strengthen the immune system and enhance the body's natural defense mechanisms.

- **Stress Relief and Relaxation:** In our fast-paced modern world, stress has become a common culprit behind many health issues. Panchakarma offers a unique opportunity to unwind, relax, and rejuvenate the body-mind complex, promoting a deep sense of relaxation and peace.

It's important to remember that panchakarma and detoxification are not just about cleansing the physical body; they are about nurturing the entire being on a holistic level. By honoring the interconnectedness of body, mind, and spirit, we can embark on a transformative journey of healing, renewal, and self-discovery.

Types of Panchakarma

There are five main types of Panchakarma therapies, each with its own unique focus and benefits. Let's explore each one in detail.

Vamana (Emesis Therapy)

Vamana is the therapeutic process of induced vomiting, primarily used to expel excess Kapha dosha from the body. This detoxification method is beneficial for those suffering from conditions related to Kapha imbalance, such as respiratory disorders, congestion, allergies, and obesity.

During Vamana, the patient is given a specific medicated drink that induces vomiting, thus eliminating toxins and excess mucus from the body. It is crucial to undergo Vamana under the supervision of a qualified Ayurvedic practitioner to ensure safety and effectiveness.

Virechana (Purgation Therapy)

Virechana involves the use of therapeutic purgation to cleanse the body of excess Pitta dosha and accumulated toxins. This cleansing process is particularly beneficial for individuals with liver disorders, skin conditions, digestive issues, and inflammation.

The patient is administered specific herbal laxatives to facilitate the elimination of waste and toxins from the intestines. Virechana helps to improve digestion, metabolism, and overall liver function, promoting balance and harmony within the body.

Basti (Enema Therapy)

Basti is a powerful therapy that focuses on balancing Vata dosha by eliminating toxins and regulating the digestive system. It involves the administration of herbal decoctions and oils through the rectum to cleanse the colon and nourish the tissues.

Basti is known for its rejuvenating and strengthening effects on the body, making it beneficial for various chronic conditions such as arthritis, constipation, neurological disorders, and reproductive health issues. The therapy helps to lubricate the intestines, remove accumulated waste, and restore balance to the body.

Nasya (Nasal Administration)

Nasya therapy involves the administration of medicated oils or herbal preparations through the nostrils to cleanse and rejuvenate the nasal passages, sinuses, and head. This therapy is useful for conditions related to the upper respiratory system, such as allergies, sinusitis, headaches, and neurological imbalances.

Nasya helps to clear congestion, improve breathing, enhance mental clarity, and promote overall relaxation. It is also beneficial for balancing the doshas in the head region and supporting optimal sensory functions.

Raktamokshana (Bloodletting Therapy)

Raktamokshana is a specialized therapy that involves the removal of impure blood from the body to eliminate toxins and balance the doshas. This ancient practice is beneficial for conditions related to blood disorders, skin diseases, and metabolic imbalances.

Raktamokshana can be performed using various methods, such as leech therapy, venesection, or using specialized tools to draw out stagnated blood. This therapy helps to improve circulation, enhance detoxification, and promote the proper function of vital organs.

Each of the five types of Panchakarma therapies plays a vital role in cleansing, rejuvenating, and restoring balance to the body according to Ayurvedic principles. By undergoing these therapies under the guidance of a knowledgeable practitioner, you can experience profound healing on physical, mental, and emotional levels.

Remember, Ayurveda views each person as a unique combination of doshas, and the Panchakarma therapies can be customized to address individual imbalances and health concerns.

Home Detox Techniques: Simple Practices for Beginners

I'm excited to share with you some simple and effective home detox techniques rooted in Ayurveda that are perfect for beginners.

So, how can you incorporate Ayurvedic detox techniques into your daily routine? Let's start with some simple practices that you can easily do at home:

- **Start Your Day with Warm Lemon Water:** Ayurveda recommends starting your day with a glass of warm water mixed with freshly squeezed lemon juice. This helps to kickstart your digestion, flush out toxins, and alkalize your body.

- **Practice Abhyanga (Self-Massage):** Treat yourself to a rejuvenating self-massage using warm, herbal oils such as sesame or coconut oil. Massage your body in long, gentle strokes before showering to promote relaxation, improve circulation, and release toxins.

- **Try Tongue Scraping:** This simple Ayurvedic practice involves using a tongue scraper to gently remove toxins and bacteria from the surface of your tongue. It not only improves oral hygiene but also enhances digestion and overall detoxification.

- **Enjoy Detoxifying Teas:** Sip on herbal teas such as ginger, turmeric, and dandelion root throughout the day to support detoxification. These teas help to stimulate digestion, support liver function, and reduce inflammation in the body.

- **Practice Mindful Eating:** Ayurveda emphasizes the importance of mindful eating to support digestion and detoxification. Take time to savor your meals, chew your food thoroughly, and avoid distractions while eating. This simple practice can have a profound impact on your overall well-being.

- **Incorporate Yoga and Pranayama:** Engage in gentle yoga postures and breathing exercises to stimulate your body's natural detoxification processes. Yoga and pranayama (breathwork) help to improve circulation, release tension, and promote the elimination of toxins from the body.

- **Dry Brushing:** Dry brushing is a popular Ayurvedic technique that involves using a dry brush to exfoliate the skin and stimulate the lymphatic system. This practice helps to remove dead skin cells, improve circulation, and support detoxification.

- **Prioritize Sleep:** Adequate rest is essential for detoxification and overall well-being. Aim to get 7-9 hours of quality sleep each night to allow your body to repair, regenerate, and eliminate toxins while you rest.

- **Mindfulness and Meditation:** Incorporate mindfulness practices and meditation into your daily routine to reduce stress, promote mental clarity, and support detoxification at a deeper level. Quieting the mind can have a powerful impact on your body's ability to detoxify.

- **Stay Hydrated:** Hydration is key to supporting your body's detoxification processes. Drink plenty of water throughout the day to flush out toxins, support digestion, and keep your body hydrated and healthy.

As you begin to incorporate these simple Ayurvedic detox techniques into your daily routine, remember to listen to your body and adjust as needed. Consistency is key when it comes to supporting your body's natural detoxification processes, so be patient and gentle with yourself as you embark on this journey to wellness.

When to Seek Professional Help: Understanding Your Limits

Now, let's delve into the importance of knowing when to seek professional assistance during your Panchakarma journey. While Ayurveda advocates self-care and self-awareness, there are certain situations where professional guidance becomes crucial for a safe and effective detoxification process.

One of the key indicators that you may need professional help is if you are experiencing severe or persistent symptoms during Panchakarma. Ayurveda teaches us to listen to our bodies and honor the signals they send us. If you find yourself struggling with intense detox reactions, physical discomfort, or emotional distress that feels overwhelming, it's time to reach out to a qualified Ayurvedic practitioner for support.

Additionally, if you have pre-existing health conditions or are taking medications, it's essential to consult with a professional before beginning Panchakarma. Certain health conditions may require modifications to the traditional detox program, and a knowledgeable practitioner can help tailor the treatment to suit your specific needs and ensure your safety throughout the process.

Moreover, seeking professional help can also be beneficial if you are new to Ayurveda or Panchakarma. A skilled practitioner can provide you with guidance on how to navigate the intricacies of this ancient healing system, offer personalized recommendations based on your unique constitution, and support you in making informed decisions for your well-being.

Now, let's shift our focus to understanding your limits while practicing Panchakarma. While the detoxification process can be incredibly rewarding, it's essential to listen to your body and honor your boundaries to prevent burnout or overwhelm.

Learning to recognize when you've reached your limit can be a valuable skill during Panchakarma. Pay attention to signs of fatigue, emotional strain, or physical discomfort, and don't hesitate to take a step back and rest when needed. Remember, self-care is an integral part of the healing journey, and it's okay to prioritize your well-being by giving yourself the time and space to recharge.

Setting realistic expectations for yourself is another crucial aspect of navigating your limits during Panchakarma. Understand that the detox process may bring up deep-seated emotions, physical challenges, or lifestyle changes that require patience and resilience. By being gentle with yourself and embracing the process with an open heart, you can cultivate a sense of balance and harmony throughout your journey.

In addition, communicating openly with your Ayurvedic practitioner about your goals, concerns, and limitations can help create a supportive environment that honors your individual needs. Together, you can work collaboratively to tailor the Panchakarma experience to align with your comfort level and ensure a positive outcome.

Chapter 6

Ayurvedic Herbs and Supplements

In Ayurveda, herbs play a pivotal role in restoring and maintaining harmony within the body, mind, and spirit. Herbs are seen as potent allies in rebalancing doshas and promoting overall well-being.

One of the key benefits of using herbs in Ayurveda is their natural and holistic approach to healing. Unlike modern medicine, which often focuses on treating symptoms, Ayurvedic herbs target the root cause of imbalances in the body. By addressing underlying issues, herbs help restore equilibrium and support the body's innate ability to heal itself.

Herbs in Ayurveda are carefully selected based on their taste, energy, and post-digestive effect, ensuring that they complement an individual's unique constitution. This personalized approach to herbal medicine highlights the importance of treating each person as an individual with distinct needs and requirements.

Another significant benefit of using herbs in Ayurveda is their gentle yet effective nature. Many Ayurvedic herbs are known for their subtle yet profound effects on the body, offering a gentle and sustainable approach to healing. Unlike harsh chemical medications, which may come with unwanted side effects, Ayurvedic herbs work in harmony with the body, promoting health and vitality without causing harm.

Furthermore, the use of herbs in Ayurveda promotes a sense of connection with nature and the environment. Ayurveda views humans as an integral part of the natural world, and herbs are seen as gifts from Mother Earth to support our well-being. By harnessing the power of plants, Ayurveda encourages a deeper appreciation for the healing properties of the natural world and fosters a sense of harmony with our surroundings.

The diverse range of herbs used in Ayurveda reflects the vast array of healing properties found in nature. From soothing herbs like chamomile and fennel to invigorating herbs like ginger and turmeric, Ayurvedic herbs offer a comprehensive toolkit for addressing a wide range of health concerns. Whether you're seeking to boost immunity, improve digestion, or calm the mind, there's an herb in Ayurveda to support your unique health goals.

One of the most fascinating aspects of Ayurvedic herbs is their ability to work synergistically with one another.

In Ayurveda, herbal formulations are often created by combining multiple herbs to enhance their therapeutic effects. This synergistic approach ensures that each herb complements the others, creating a powerful blend that addresses multiple aspects of a health issue.

Ayurvedic herbs are not only used internally but also externally in the form of oils, ointments, and poultices. This holistic approach to herbal medicine acknowledges the importance of treating the body both internally and externally to promote optimal health and well-being. Whether applied topically or ingested, Ayurvedic herbs offer a versatile and comprehensive approach to healing.

Furthermore, Ayurvedic herbs are often used in conjunction with other holistic practices, such as yoga, meditation, and pranayama (breathwork). This integrated approach to wellness recognizes the interconnectedness of the body, mind, and spirit and emphasizes the importance of maintaining balance in all aspects of life. By incorporating herbs into a holistic wellness routine, individuals can enhance their overall health and vitality on multiple levels.

Now that you know why herbs are fantastic to add to your Ayurvedic practice, let's take a look at some of the most commonly used ones.

Common Ayurvedic Herbs

The natural world is huge, so it shouldn't be a surprise that there are countless herbs you can incorporate into your Ayurvedic practice. However, the ten most commonly used ones are:

- Ashwagandha (Withania somnifera)
- Turmeric (Curcuma longa)
- Triphala (a combination of three fruits: Amalaki, Bibhitaki, and Haritaki)
- Tulsi (Ocimum sanctum, also known as Holy Basil)
- Brahmi (Bacopa monnieri)
- Ginger (Zingiber officinale)
- Amla (Emblica officinalis, also known as Indian Gooseberry)
- Neem (Azadirachta indica)
- Guggul (Commiphora wightii)
- Licorice (Glycyrrhiza glabra)

Let's take a detailed look at each one.

Ashwagandha

Ashwagandha, also known as "Indian Winter Cherry" or "Indian Ginseng," is a powerful herb that has been revered in Ayurvedic medicine for thousands of years. Its botanical name, Withania somnifera, reflects its potent rejuvenating and restorative properties.

This herb is believed to embody the characteristics of a warrior: strong, resilient, and adaptable. Just like a warrior, Ashwagandha helps to combat stress, improve vitality, and enhance overall well-being. It is known for its unique ability to balance all three doshas – Vata, Pitta, and Kapha – making it a versatile herb suited for a wide range of individuals.

In Ayurveda, Ashwagandha is classified as a rasayana, which is a category of herbs that promote longevity, vitality, and overall health. It is particularly revered for its adaptogenic properties, which means it helps the body adapt to stress and maintain homeostasis.

One of the key benefits of Ashwagandha is its ability to support the nervous system. In Ayurveda, it is considered a medhya herb, which means it enhances cognitive function and promotes mental clarity. Ashwagandha is known to calm the mind, reduce anxiety, and promote restful sleep, making it an invaluable herb for those dealing with stress and insomnia.

Ashwagandha is also renowned for its rejuvenating effects on the body. It is believed to strengthen the immune system, increase vitality, and improve overall energy levels. This makes it a valuable herb for individuals looking to boost their resilience and endurance.

From a personality standpoint, Ashwagandha can be likened to a wise sage, full of ancient knowledge and profound insights. It imparts a sense of groundedness and stability, helping individuals connect to their inner strength and wisdom. Just like a sage, Ashwagandha guides individuals on a path towards holistic well-being and balance.

In Ayurveda, Ashwagandha is often recommended for individuals with high Vata imbalances, such as anxiety, restlessness, and insomnia. Its grounding and nourishing properties help to pacify excess Vata and bring about a sense of calm and stability.

Ashwagandha's warming and nourishing qualities make it beneficial for individuals with high Pitta imbalances as well. It helps to soothe inflammation, support the adrenal glands, and promote a sense of coolness and balance in the body.

For those with high Kapha imbalances, Ashwagandha's stimulating and rejuvenating properties can help invigorate the mind and body. It helps to increase energy levels, improve digestion, and uplift the spirits, making it a valuable herb for individuals dealing with lethargy and heaviness.

Incorporating Ashwagandha into your daily routine can bring about a sense of vitality, resilience, and balance. Whether you're looking to combat stress, improve cognitive function, or enhance your overall well-being, this herb has much to offer.

Just like a trusted companion, Ashwagandha guides you on a journey towards optimal health and vitality, supporting you every step of the way. Embrace the wisdom of this ancient herb and experience its transformative effects on your mind, body, and spirit. Ashwagandha truly is a gift from nature, a warrior herb standing strong and resilient, ready to support you in your quest for well-being.

Turmeric

Turmeric, the golden spice of Ayurveda, is truly a gem in the world of holistic health and wellness. Vibrant in color and rich in history, this potent herb has been prized for centuries for its numerous health benefits.

Imagine walking through a bustling market in ancient India, where the aroma of freshly ground spices fills the air. Among the myriad of herbs and spices, turmeric stands out with its bright yellow hue, beckoning you to experience its magical properties. In Ayurveda, turmeric is classified as "kapha-pacifying," helping to balance the earth and water elements in the body. It is known to possess warming energy, promote circulation, and assist in the digestion of heavy foods.

Turmeric is revered for its ability to pacify all three doshas: Vata, Pitta, and Kapha. It is a true all-rounder that can adapt to the unique needs of each individual, making it a versatile herb in Ayurvedic medicine. Turmeric's bitter and pungent taste works to stimulate digestion, cleanse the blood, and support healthy liver function. It is also a powerful anti-inflammatory agent, making it invaluable for those dealing with joint pain and inflammation.

In terms of energetics, turmeric carries the qualities of being light, dry, and heating. It kindles the digestive fire, known as "Agni" in Ayurveda, helping to improve metabolism and support the body's natural detoxification processes. This makes turmeric an essential ingredient in traditional Ayurvedic cooking, where it is used in curries, dals, and medicinal teas.

Beyond its culinary uses, turmeric is also a star player in Ayurvedic skincare and beauty rituals. Its antioxidant and anti-inflammatory properties make it a wonderful remedy for acne, eczema, and other skin conditions. A paste made from turmeric and honey can work wonders for brightening the complexion and promoting healthy, radiant skin.

Turmeric's benefits extend beyond the physical realm, as it is also revered for its mental and spiritual properties. In Ayurveda, turmeric is said to have a purifying effect on the mind, helping to clear away mental fog and promote clarity of thought. Its warm and invigorating energy can uplift the spirits and promote a sense of well-being.

To incorporate turmeric into your daily routine, you can start by adding it to your cooking. A sprinkle of turmeric in soups, stews, and roasted vegetables can enhance both the flavor and health benefits of your meals. You can also enjoy a soothing cup of turmeric tea by steeping freshly grated turmeric in hot water with a dash of honey and lemon.

For those looking to harness the full power of turmeric, Ayurveda offers various formulations and remedies. Turmeric capsules, powders, and oils are widely available and can be used to address specific health concerns. Whether you are looking to support joint health, boost immunity, or improve digestion, turmeric has something to offer for everyone.

Triphala

Triphala is considered one of the most revered herbal formulations in Ayurveda, the ancient Indian system of medicine that focuses on balancing the body, mind, and spirit to achieve optimal health. This powerful combination of three fruits, Amla (Emblica officinalis), Haritaki (Terminalia chebula), and Bibhitaki (Terminalia belerica), has been used for centuries to promote overall well-being and longevity.

Picture Triphala as a dynamic trio of Ayurvedic superheroes, each fruit bringing its own unique strengths to the table. Amla, also known as Indian gooseberry, is a powerhouse of vitamin C and antioxidants. It rejuvenates the body and enhances immunity, like a resilient shield protecting you from illnesses. Haritaki, the gentle cleanser, supports digestive health and detoxification, ensuring that your internal systems run smoothly like a well-oiled machine. Finally, Bibhitaki, the balancer, promotes respiratory health and helps to maintain equilibrium in the body, mind, and spirit, akin to a wise counselor keeping everything in harmony.

Triphala, with its holistic approach, addresses a wide range of health issues and is known for its gentle yet effective nature. It supports healthy digestion, relieves constipation, and detoxifies the body, making it a cornerstone for good gastrointestinal health. Think of it as a gentle broom sweeping away toxins and debris, leaving your digestive system clean and rejuvenated.

But Triphala's benefits don't stop there. It also nourishes the eyes, hair, and skin, promoting a radiant appearance from within. It's like a beauty elixir that works on enhancing your outer glow by nourishing your inner vitality. Triphala's antioxidant properties help to combat free radicals, which are often the culprit behind premature aging and various health issues.

Furthermore, Triphala has a unique ability to support weight management by balancing the three Doshas – Vata, Pitta, and Kapha – in the body. It aids in metabolism, digestion, and elimination, promoting a healthy weight and overall well-being. Triphala doesn't believe in crash diets or quick fixes; it's all about sustainable and balanced health that lasts a lifetime.

When it comes to mental well-being, Triphala shines as a rejuvenator for the mind. It helps to alleviate stress, improve cognitive function, and enhance clarity and focus. Imagine having a calm and focused mind, free from the chaos and clutter of everyday life, thanks to the balancing effects of Triphala.

Tulsi

Tulsi, also known as Holy Basil, is a beloved herb in Ayurveda, celebrated for its numerous healing properties and sacred significance. With a personality as vibrant and invigorating as its aroma, Tulsi is often referred to as the "Queen of Herbs" due to its exceptional adaptogenic qualities.

In Ayurveda, Tulsi is classified as a sattvic herb, known for its ability to balance all three doshas (Vata, Pitta, and Kapha). With its bitter and pungent taste, Tulsi helps pacify Kapha dosha, while its warming qualities aid in soothing Vata imbalance. Additionally, its cooling properties make it beneficial for Pitta dosha, making it a versatile herb for promoting overall well-being.

Tulsi is rich in essential oils, vitamins, and minerals, making it a potent herb for boosting the immune system and improving resilience to stress. Its adaptogenic properties help the body adapt to physical, emotional, and environmental stressors, promoting a sense of balance and harmony.

When it comes to personality, Tulsi is known for its nurturing and protective nature. Just like a caring mother, it offers support and strength during challenging times, helping individuals navigate through life's ups and downs with grace and resilience. Tulsi exudes a sense of calm and serenity, providing a sanctuary of peace amidst life's chaos.

Tulsi is often used in Ayurvedic medicine to treat a wide range of health conditions. It is considered a potent rasayana, or rejuvenating herb, that helps promote longevity and vitality. Tulsi is known for its antimicrobial properties, making it effective in treating respiratory infections, coughs, and colds. Its anti-inflammatory properties help reduce inflammation in the body, making it a valuable herb for managing conditions like arthritis and inflammatory bowel diseases.

As a powerful antioxidant, Tulsi helps protect the body from damaging free radicals, reducing the risk of chronic diseases and premature aging. Its detoxifying properties support liver function, aiding in the elimination of toxins from the body. Tulsi is also known for its beneficial effects on the nervous system, helping improve cognitive function, memory, and mental clarity.

In Ayurveda, Tulsi is not just a medicinal herb but also a spiritual ally. It is revered for its purifying and calming influence on the mind and spirit. Tulsi is often used in rituals and ceremonies to enhance spiritual awareness and connection with the divine. Its subtle yet profound energy helps create a sacred space for meditation and inner reflection.

Brahmi

Nestled in the lush greenery of the Indian subcontinent, Brahmi, also known as Bacopa monnieri, has long been celebrated as a powerful adaptogen and cognitive enhancer in Ayurvedic tradition.

In Ayurveda, Brahmi is revered for its ability to pacify all three doshas - Vata, Pitta, and Kapha, making it a versatile herb suitable for almost everyone. Its cooling and grounding qualities soothe fiery Pitta imbalances, while its nourishing essence calms restless Vata energies. At the same time, it gently balances the heavy qualities of Kapha, bringing a sense of lightness and clarity to the mind and body.

Brahmi is particularly cherished for its impact on the intellect and mental function. Known as a Medhya Rasayana in Ayurveda, it is believed to enhance cognitive abilities, memory, and overall brain health. Imagine Brahmi as a wise sage whispering ancient secrets to your mind, enhancing your learning and comprehension with each passing day.

The herb's profound effects on the mind extend to its ability to calm the nervous system and promote mental clarity. In a world filled with distractions and stress, Brahmi acts as a soothing balm, helping you find inner peace and focus amidst the chaos. It gently uplifts the mood, easing anxiety and promoting a sense of tranquility that lingers like a sweet melody in your soul.

But Brahmi's benefits do not stop at the mind. Its rejuvenating properties also extend to the physical body, nourishing the tissues and supporting overall vitality. Imagine your body as a temple, with Brahmi as the gentle caretaker, tending to every cell and organ with love and devotion.

As you welcome Brahmi into your wellness routine, you may notice an increase in energy, stamina, and resilience. Like a gentle breeze that revitalizes the spirit, Brahmi infuses your being with a newfound sense of vitality and strength, enabling you to navigate life's challenges with grace and poise.

In Ayurvedic terms, Brahmi is said to enhance Ojas, the subtle essence of vitality and immunity. By bolstering your body's natural defenses, Brahmi acts as a shield against environmental stressors and imbalances, helping you maintain optimal health and well-being throughout the year.

So, as you sip on a cup of Brahmi tea or add a few drops of its herbal extract to your daily routine, remember the wisdom and grace of this extraordinary herb. Let Brahmi be your guiding light in the journey towards balance and harmony, a steadfast companion on the path to radiant health and vibrant vitality.

Ginger

Ginger, known as "shunthi" in Sanskrit, has been a beloved herb in Ayurvedic medicine for centuries, appreciated for its warming properties and ability to balance the body's doshas – Vata, Pitta, and Kapha. This knobby rhizome, with its unique blend of flavors, holds a special place in Ayurveda as a versatile herb that can be used in cooking, teas, and medicinal remedies. Just like a fiery personality, ginger leaves a lasting impression wherever it goes.

In Ayurveda, ginger is particularly respected for its digestive properties. It enhances the digestive fire, or "agni," aiding in the proper digestion and assimilation of food. A cup of warm ginger tea after meals can help soothe any lingering digestive discomfort, promoting a sense of lightness and balance in the stomach. It's like a warm hug for your belly after a hearty meal!

From an Ayurvedic perspective, ginger is known to pacify Vata and Kapha doshas while potentially aggravating Pitta when consumed in excess. This makes it a wonderful herb for balancing the cold and damp qualities of winter or calming an anxious mind, all while offering a spicy kick of flavor to awaken the senses. Like a trustworthy friend, Ginger is always there to provide comfort and support when needed.

In addition to its digestive benefits, ginger is also revered for its anti-inflammatory properties. This makes it a popular choice in Ayurvedic treatments for conditions like arthritis and muscle pain. Its warming nature helps to improve circulation and reduce inflammation, providing relief to those with achy joints and muscles. Ginger's ability to ignite a gentle fire within the body can help melt away tension and stiffness, leaving you feeling rejuvenated and invigorated.

Furthermore, ginger is celebrated for its immune-boosting qualities. Rich in antioxidants and antimicrobial compounds, ginger can help strengthen the body's defense mechanisms against pathogens and infections. A soothing ginger and honey concoction is often used in Ayurveda to alleviate cold and flu symptoms, offering natural relief that tickles the taste buds and warms the soul.

The versatility of ginger extends beyond medicinal uses, as it can also be incorporated into daily cooking to enhance both the flavor and health benefits of a dish. Whether grated, sliced, or juiced, ginger adds a zesty touch to curries, stir-fries, soups, and desserts, infusing each bite with its spicy-sweet essence.

Amla

Meet Amla, the ancient Indian superfruit known for its incredible health benefits and powerful impact on overall well-being. Amla, also known as Indian Gooseberry, has been revered in Ayurveda for thousands of years as a symbol of good health, longevity, and vitality.

With its sour and bitter taste, Amla contains a high concentration of Vitamin C, making it one of the richest natural sources of this essential nutrient. This powerful antioxidant helps boost the immune system, promote healthy skin, and support the body in fighting off illness and disease. Amla is also a potent source of bioflavonoids, which work synergistically with Vitamin C to enhance its effects and provide a wide range of health benefits.

In Ayurveda, Amla is considered a "rasayana" herb, which means it is believed to promote longevity, rejuvenation, and overall vitality. This makes Amla an essential component of many Ayurvedic formulations and remedies aimed at restoring balance to the body and mind.

Amla is known for its ability to support digestion and enhance nutrient absorption. It helps balance the digestive fire, known as "agni" in Ayurveda, which is essential for proper digestion and metabolism. Amla's bitter and sour taste stimulates digestive enzymes and promotes the breakdown of food, helping to prevent indigestion, bloating, and other digestive issues.

Not only does Amla support digestion, but it also acts as a natural detoxifier for the body. It helps cleanse the liver and kidneys, promoting the elimination of toxins and waste products from the body. This detoxifying action helps improve overall health and well-being, leaving you feeling lighter, more energetic and rejuvenated.

Amla is also known for its anti-inflammatory properties, making it an excellent remedy for inflammatory conditions such as arthritis, joint pain, and skin disorders. Its cooling and soothing nature helps reduce inflammation and provide relief from pain and discomfort.

But Amla's benefits extend beyond just physical health; it is also known for its impact on mental and emotional well-being. In Ayurveda, Amla is considered a "medhya" herb, which means it is believed to support cognitive function, memory, and concentration. Its nourishing qualities help calm the mind, reduce stress and anxiety, and promote mental clarity and focus.

Amla is truly a versatile superfruit that can be consumed in various forms: fresh, dried, powdered, or as a juice. It can be incorporated into your diet in countless ways, from adding it to smoothies and salads to brewing it as a tea or tonic. However, you choose to enjoy Amla, rest assured that you are nourishing your body, mind, and spirit with this ancient Ayurvedic gem.

Neem

Neem, also known as Azadirachta indica, is hailed as the "village pharmacy" in India for its wide array of health benefits. This evergreen tree is native to the Indian subcontinent and has been revered for centuries for its medicinal qualities. Neem is considered a symbol of good health and protection, earning it the nickname "the divine tree."

One of the key characteristics of Neem is its bitter taste, which is a reflection of its powerful purifying properties. In Ayurveda, this bitter taste is associated with reducing excess Kapha and Pitta doshas, making Neem an excellent herb for balancing these doshas in the body. Its cleansing and detoxifying effects make it a popular choice for promoting healthy skin, supporting liver function, and aiding digestion.

Neem is a powerhouse of active compounds such as nimbin, nimbidin, and nimbidol, which contribute to its antimicrobial, antifungal, and anti-inflammatory properties. These compounds work together to combat a wide range of health issues, from skin infections and acne to digestive disorders and immune system support.

As the ultimate skin savior, Neem is known for its ability to cleanse, moisturize, and rejuvenate the skin. Its antibacterial and antifungal properties make it a popular ingredient in skincare products for treating acne, eczema, and other skin conditions. Neem oil, derived from the seeds of the Neem tree, is a potent remedy for promoting healthy skin and hair, thanks to its nourishing and protective effects.

In addition to its skincare benefits, Neem is also a versatile herb for promoting overall well-being. It is commonly used in Ayurvedic remedies for supporting healthy blood sugar levels, boosting immunity, and even as a natural insect repellent. Neem leaves are often consumed as a tea or added to dishes for their detoxifying and immune-boosting effects.

Neem's influence extends beyond physical health to spiritual and mental well-being. This herb is believed to have a purifying and protective energy that wards off negative influences and promotes spiritual growth. Adding Neem to your daily routine can help create a sense of balance and harmony within the body, mind, and spirit.

Neem, with its bitter taste and potent properties, may not be the most popular herb in the world of Ayurveda, but its benefits are truly remarkable. From skin care to immune support, this versatile herb has a lot to offer for those seeking natural remedies for their health and well-being.

Guggul

Guggul is a resin-like no other, revered in the realms of Ayurveda for its potent healing properties and age-old wisdom. Picture a tree standing tall and strong in the mystical lands of India, its resin oozing out like liquid gold, holding within it the secrets of wellness and vitality.

In the ancient texts of Ayurveda, guggul shines as a superstar remedy, known for its ability to balance all three doshas - Vata, Pitta, and Kapha. It's like a harmonious orchestra conductor, bringing your body and mind back into perfect rhythm. A true all-rounder, guggul is beloved for its versatile nature, effectively addressing a myriad of health concerns.

When it comes to Ayurvedic energetics, guggul's taste profile is pungent, bitter, and astringent, with a warming potency that kindles your digestive fire. As it journeys through your system, it penetrates deeply, detoxifying and purifying at a cellular level. Guggul's post-digestive effect is sweet, leaving a soothing touch as it replenishes and nurtures your tissues.

Guggul's primary action lies in its profound ability to support healthy cholesterol levels and promote cardiovascular wellness. It's like a loyal guardian, standing sentinel against the buildup of plaque and ensuring your heart beats harmoniously. But Guggul doesn't stop there - oh no! This benevolent resin is also known for its anti-inflammatory prowess and soothing joints and muscles, making movement a joy once more.

As we delve deeper into guggul's realm, we uncover its talent for kindling the digestive flames, aiding in metabolism and weight management. It's like a whisper from the ancient sages, guiding you towards balance and vitality. Guggul's purifying nature extends to the liver, supporting its detoxification functions and promoting radiant skin from within.

But wait, there's more! Guggul's influence on the respiratory system is nothing short of magical. Like a breath of fresh air on a misty morning, it clears congestion, eases breathing, and uplifts your spirits. It's the gentle hand that guides you towards clarity and lightness, one inhalation at a time.

And let's not forget Guggul's impact on the mind. This resin holds a special place in Ayurvedic tradition for its ability to pacify the mind, calm the nerves, and uplift the spirit. It's like a wise old friend, offering solace in times of turbulence and clarity in moments of confusion.

Licorice

Licorice, also known as "Yashtimadhu" in Ayurvedic texts, is a herb with a rich history of medicinal use in various cultures. In Ayurveda, Licorice is classified as a "Rasayana" herb, which means it is renowned for its rejuvenating properties. This herb holds a special place in Ayurvedic pharmacology for its ability to balance all three doshas: Vata, Pitta, and Kapha. Licorice is particularly beneficial for Pitta dosha imbalances, as it helps to cool and soothe excess heat in the body.

One of the key characteristics of Licorice is its sweet taste, which is attributed to the compound glycyrrhizin. This natural sweetness makes Licorice a delightful addition to herbal formulations, balancing out the bitter and pungent tastes of other herbs. The sweet taste of Licorice also has a nourishing and grounding effect on the body and mind, making it a wonderful choice for promoting overall well-being.

Licorice is revered for its adaptogenic properties, which means it helps the body adapt to stress and maintain a state of homeostasis. This makes Licorice a valuable herb for supporting the body during times of physical or emotional stress. From supporting the adrenal glands to promoting healthy digestion, Licorice works holistically to keep the body in balance.

When it comes to digestion, Licorice is a true superstar. This herb is known for its ability to soothe the digestive tract, relieve gastrointestinal discomfort, and support healthy bowel movements. Licorice can help alleviate symptoms of indigestion, bloating, and heartburn, making it a go-to remedy for maintaining gut health.

Licorice also boasts powerful antioxidant properties, helping to protect the body from oxidative stress and free radical damage. By neutralizing harmful molecules in the body, Licorice promotes cellular health and overall vitality. This herb is a true ally in the fight against premature aging and disease, keeping you feeling vibrant and youthful from the inside out.

In addition to its physical benefits, Licorice has a calming effect on the mind and emotions. This herb is traditionally used in Ayurveda to promote mental clarity, emotional balance, and a sense of inner peace. Licorice can help reduce feelings of stress and anxiety, bringing a sense of calm and tranquility to the mind.

Licorice is a versatile herb that can be enjoyed in various forms, including teas, powders, and syrups. Whether you sip on a cup of Licorice tea to soothe a sore throat or incorporate Licorice powder into your cooking for digestive support, this herb is easy to incorporate into your daily routine.

Making Herbal Preparations: Teas, Tinctures, and Powders

Making herbal preparations in Ayurveda is as delightful as it is beneficial for both the body and the soul. From teas to tinctures and powders, there's a wide array of methods to harness the power of nature's pharmacy.

Let's start with the basics: teas. Herbal teas are not only a soothing and fragrant way to enjoy the benefits of herbs, but they also provide a gentle way to introduce the healing properties of herbs into your daily routine. To make a calming and balancing herbal tea, try this recipe:

Soothing Balance Tea

Ingredients:

- 1 tsp dried chamomile flowers
- 1 tsp dried lavender flowers
- 1 tsp dried rose petals
- 1 tsp dried lemon balm
- 2 cups of water

Instructions:

1. Boil the water in a saucepan.
2. Add the dried herbs to the boiling water.
3. Cover and let steep for 10–15 minutes.
4. Strain the herbs and enjoy your soothing balance tea.

Next up, tinctures. Tinctures are concentrated liquid extracts of herbs that preserve their medicinal properties. They are easy to make and convenient to take. Try this recipe for an energizing and immune-boosting tincture:

Immune Boost Tincture

Ingredients:

- 1 part echinacea root
- 1 part astragalus root
- 1 part ginger root
- Vodka or brandy

Instructions:

- Chop the roots into small pieces.
- Place the herbs in a glass jar and cover with the alcohol.
- Shake the jar daily and let it infuse for 4-6 weeks.
- Strain the tincture and store it in a dark glass bottle.
- Take 1-2 droppers full daily to boost your immune system.

Lastly, let's talk about powders. Herbal powders are versatile and can be easily incorporated into smoothies, teas, or capsules. They are a convenient way to consume a potent dose of herbs. Here is a recipe for a grounding and nourishing herbal powder:

Nourishing Ashwagandha Powder

Ingredients:

- 1/2 cup ashwagandha root powder
- 1/4 cup cinnamon powder
- 1/4 cup cardamom powder

Instructions:

1. Mix all the powders together in a bowl.
2. Store the powder in an airtight container.
3. Add a teaspoon of the powder to your morning smoothie or warm milk for a nourishing boost.

In Ayurveda, every herb has specific healing properties that can be utilized to restore balance and harmony to the body. Experiment with different herbs and preparations to find what works best for you. Remember, herbal preparations are not only meant to heal the body but also to nourish the spirit. Embrace the process of creating these herbal remedies as a form of self-care and self-love.

Now, how about a couple more recipes to add to your herbal repertoire?

Digestive Tea Blend

Ingredients:

- 1 tsp fennel seeds

- 1 tsp coriander seeds
- 1 tsp cumin seeds
- 2 cups of water

Instructions:

1. Toast the seeds in a dry pan until fragrant.
2. Crush the seeds slightly to release their aroma.
3. Boil the water and add the seeds.
4. Let steep for 10 minutes, strain, and enjoy after meals for better digestion.

Calming Lavender Tincture

Ingredients:

- 1 part dried lavender flowers
- Vodka or brandy

Instructions:

- Place the dried lavender flowers in a glass jar.
- Cover with alcohol and let it infuse for 4-6 weeks.
- Strain the tincture and store it in a dark glass bottle.
- Take a dropper full before bed for a restful night's sleep.

Remember to have fun, be creative, and let the healing power of herbs guide you on your journey to wellness.

Safety and Dosage: Guidelines for Using Herbs Responsibly

When it comes to dosage, the golden rule in Ayurveda is moderation. It is always advisable to start with a lower dose and gradually increase it as needed, allowing your body to adjust and respond to the herb's effects. Consulting with a qualified Ayurvedic practitioner can provide valuable insights into the appropriate dosage for your specific condition and constitution, ensuring a safe and harmonious healing journey.

In addition to dosage, the quality and purity of the herbs you use play a crucial role in their safety and efficacy. Opt for organic, sustainably sourced herbs from reputable suppliers, and avoid herbs that are contaminated with pesticides, heavy metals, or other harmful substances. Ayurveda emphasizes the importance of honoring the integrity of nature and choosing products that are in harmony with the environment and our well-being.

As with any form of medicine, it is essential to be mindful of potential interactions between herbs and other medications you may be taking. Some herbs can interfere with the effectiveness of certain drugs or exacerbate underlying health conditions, so it is advisable to inform your healthcare provider about your herbal regimen to ensure compatibility and safety.

To enhance the absorption and effectiveness of herbs, Ayurveda offers various preparation methods, such as decoctions, powders, and oils. Each method has its own unique benefits and can be tailored to suit your preferences and needs. Experimenting with different preparations can add a delightful dimension to your herbal journey and enhance the therapeutic effects of the herbs you choose.

In the vast and enchanting realm of Ayurveda, safety, and dosage are paramount considerations that guide us in harnessing the healing power of herbs. By approaching herbs with respect, wisdom, and an open heart, we can unlock their full potential and embark on a transformative path towards well-being and balance.

Chapter 7

Ayurvedic Bodywork and Self-Care

Imagine you are surrounded by the soothing scent of essential oils, soft music playing in the background, and warm herbal oils being gently massaged into your skin. This is the magic of Ayurvedic bodywork, where every touch is intentional and every movement is designed to restore balance to your unique constitution, or dosha.

But Ayurvedic self-care is not just about the treatments you receive from a practitioner; it's also about the practices you incorporate into your daily routine to maintain that sense of balance and well-being. From self-massage with nourishing oils to practicing mindfulness and meditation, Ayurvedic self-care empowers you to take charge of your health and wellness in a holistic way.

In this chapter, we'll explore methods to ensure you're getting all the self-care you need in your Ayurvedic endeavors.

Abhyanga (Self-Massage)

Abhyanga, the ancient practice of self-massage in Ayurveda, is a luxurious and nurturing ritual that offers a host of physical, mental, and emotional benefits. This beautiful practice involves lovingly anointing the body with warm oil, allowing it to penetrate deep into the skin and tissues, and then gently massaging the body to promote relaxation, balance, and overall well-being.

Let's start by exploring the many benefits of abhyanga. First and foremost, abhyanga helps to nourish and moisturize the skin, leaving it soft, supple, and radiant. The warm oil used in abhyanga also helps to improve circulation, boosting the flow of nutrients and oxygen throughout the body. This can help to reduce muscle tension, alleviate aches and pains, and promote overall relaxation. In addition, abhyanga is believed to support the lymphatic system, helping to detoxify the body and boost the immune system.

On a mental and emotional level, abhyanga is a deeply grounding and soothing practice. The act of massaging the body with warm oil can help to calm the mind, reduce stress and anxiety, and promote a sense of inner peace. The rhythmic motions of the massage can help to release emotional tension stored in the body, allowing you to feel more balanced and centered. In Ayurveda, it is believed that abhyanga helps to balance the doshas, or the unique elemental energies within each individual, leading to improved overall health and well-being.

Now, let's dive into some techniques for performing an abhyanga self-massage ritual. To begin, choose a high-quality oil that is appropriate for your dosha or current imbalances. Warm the oil slightly by placing the bottle in a bowl of warm water or by using a gentle heating method. Start by standing on a towel or mat in a warm room, as you want to be comfortable and relaxed during the massage.

Begin by applying a small amount of oil to your scalp, massaging it into the roots of your hair using circular motions. Then, move on to your face and ears, using gentle upward strokes to nourish and rejuvenate the delicate skin. Next, massage your neck and shoulders, using long, soothing strokes to release tension and stress. Move down to your arms and hands, paying special attention to the joints and muscles that may hold tension.

As you move to your chest and abdomen, use gentle circular motions to promote digestion and release emotional tension stored in the solar plexus area. Continue down to your legs and feet, massaging each muscle and joint with care and attention. Take your time with each part of your body, allowing the warm oil and loving touch to penetrate deeply and nourish your entire being.

After you have completed the massage, take a warm bath or shower to further enhance the benefits of the oil. Allow the water to cleanse and rejuvenate your body, leaving you feeling refreshed and renewed. Pat your skin dry with a soft towel, taking a few moments to bask in the glow of your self-care ritual.

Remember, abhyanga is a practice of self-love and self-care, so be gentle and kind to yourself throughout the process. Allow yourself to fully experience the nurturing touch of the oil and the healing power of your own hands. You deserve this time to reconnect with your body, mind, and spirit and to honor the ancient wisdom of Ayurveda.

Shirodhara: Oil Pouring Therapy for Stress Relief

Are you feeling overwhelmed by the hustle and bustle of daily life? Are stress and anxiety creeping in, making it difficult to find your inner calm? Well, fear not, because Shirodhara will have you feeling like you're floating on cloud nine in no time!

Shirodhara, derived from the Sanskrit words "Shiro" (head) and "Dhara" (flow), is a traditional Ayurvedic therapy that involves the continuous and gentle pouring of warm herbal oil over the forehead and scalp. This deeply relaxing treatment is not just about pampering yourself; it's a holistic approach to healing and rejuvenation that can help alleviate stress, anxiety, insomnia, and a myriad of other health issues.

Picture this: you're lying down on a comfortable massage table, soft music playing in the background, as a skilled therapist begins to pour a stream of warm, herb-infused oil onto your forehead in a rhythmic motion. The oil flows gently over your scalp, creating a sensation of pure bliss as it penetrates deep into your nervous system, soothing your mind and calming your senses.

One of the key principles of Ayurveda is the belief that our physical, mental, and emotional well-being are interconnected. When stress and tension build up in our bodies, it can manifest in a variety of ways, from headaches and muscle stiffness to digestive issues and insomnia. Shirodhara works by balancing the subtle energies within the body, promoting relaxation, and enhancing the body's natural healing processes.

The benefits of Shirodhara extend far beyond just stress relief. This therapeutic practice is known to improve mental clarity, enhance concentration, and promote a sense of inner peace and well-being. By calming the mind and soothing the nervous system, Shirodhara can also help improve sleep quality, boost immunity, and promote overall vitality and longevity.

But what sets Shirodhara apart from other relaxation techniques is its ability to induce a state of deep meditation and promote a profound sense of inner transformation. As the warm oil cascades over your forehead, it can help quiet the chatter of the mind, creating a space for introspection and self-discovery. Many people who have experienced Shirodhara report feeling a deep sense of clarity, insight, and emotional release during the treatment.

Of course, it's not possible to perform Shirodhara on yourself, but you could perform it on someone else. Here's how:

- **Set the scene:** Create a peaceful and calming atmosphere in the room where you will be performing Shirodhara. Dim the lights, play soft instrumental music, and light some aromatic candles or incense to enhance the experience.
- **Choose the right oil:** Select a high-quality, warm oil such as sesame, coconut, or almond oil for your Shirodhara treatment. Warm the oil gently in a double boiler or a bowl placed in hot water until it reaches a comfortable temperature.
- **Position the recipient:** Have the person receiving the treatment lie down on a comfortable surface with their head supported by a small pillow. Place a towel or plastic sheet under their head to catch any excess oil.

- **Begin the pour:** Using a special vessel called a Shirodhara pot or a simple container with a small hole in the bottom, start pouring the warm oil in a steady stream over the center of the person's forehead, just above the eyebrows. Adjust the flow of oil to a gentle and consistent stream.

- **Relax and rejuvenate:** Encourage the recipient to close their eyes, take deep breaths, and surrender to the soothing sensation of the warm oil cascading over their forehead. Let the oil flow for 20–30 minutes, allowing them to drift into a state of deep relaxation.

- **End with a scalp massage:** After the Shirodhara session, gently massage the scalp and neck to help further relax the muscles and promote circulation. Allow the recipient to rest for a few minutes before they slowly rise from the treatment.

Marma Therapy: The Art of Energy Point Massage

Marma massage, also known as energy point massage, is a traditional Indian healing technique that focuses on stimulating specific points in the body to promote physical, emotional, and spiritual well-being. These energy points, known as Marma points, are believed to be junctures where two or more types of tissue meet, such as muscles, veins, ligaments, or bones, and are considered vital energy centers within the body.

The origins of Marma massage date back thousands of years to ancient Indian healing traditions, where it was used as a form of medicine to restore balance and the flow of energy within the body. Marma points are believed to be closely connected to the body's energy channels, or nadis, through which prana, or life force, flows. By stimulating these points through massage, practitioners aim to remove blockages, improve energy flow, and restore harmony to the body and mind.

To perform Marma massage, it is important to have a clear understanding of the location and significance of the Marma points on the body. There are said to be 107 major Marma points, with each point having its own unique properties and effects on the body. Some Marma points are considered more vital than others and require special care and attention when massaging.

Before beginning a Marma massage session, it is essential to create a peaceful and calming environment to help the recipient relax and fully benefit from the treatment. Soft lighting, soothing music, and the use of essential oils can enhance the overall experience and promote a sense of tranquility. It is also important to establish a connection with the recipient and ensure open communication throughout the massage session.

To perform Marma massage, start by applying a small amount of warm oil to the hands to create a smooth and lubricated surface for massaging. Begin by gently massaging the recipient's body with long, smooth strokes to help relax the muscles and prepare the body for the more targeted Marma point stimulation.

Once the recipient is relaxed, gently palpate the Marma points using light pressure and circular motions to awaken the energy centers. Focus on each Marma point individually, paying attention to any areas of tenderness or sensitivity. Use your intuition and expertise to determine the appropriate amount of pressure and duration for each point based on the recipient's needs and comfort level.

As you stimulate the Marma points, encourage the recipient to take slow, deep breaths to help facilitate the flow of energy throughout the body. Pay attention to the recipient's reactions and adjust your technique accordingly to ensure a comfortable and effective massage experience.

Incorporating different massage techniques such as kneading, tapping, and vibration can help enhance the effects of Marma massage and promote relaxation, stress relief, and overall well-being. Be mindful of the recipient's feedback and adapt your approach to address any areas of tension or discomfort.

Throughout the massage session, maintain a sense of presence and mindfulness to create a sacred space for healing and rejuvenation. Express genuine care and compassion for the recipient and convey positive energy through your touch and intention.

After completing the Marma massage, allow the recipient time to rest and integrate the experience. Offer a warm cup of herbal tea or water to help hydrate and ground the body. Encourage the recipient to reflect on their experience and notice any changes or sensations that arise following the treatment.

Integrating Self-Care Practices

Ayurveda is not just a system of medicine; it's a way of life that promotes holistic well-being. Within that, self-care is vital.

Daily self-care routines in Ayurveda focus on setting a harmonious rhythm for your day, starting with a morning routine called Dinacharya. This routine is tailored to balance your dosha. We already mentioned a few morning routines you can try within this, but let's quickly refresh your memory:

- **Tongue scraping:** Your tongue accumulates toxins overnight, and tongue scraping helps remove these toxins for better oral hygiene and digestion.
- **Oil pulling:** Swishing coconut or sesame oil in your mouth for a few minutes helps detoxify and freshen your breath.

- **Dry brushing:** Use a natural bristle brush to stimulate circulation and exfoliate dead skin cells, promoting healthy skin.
- **Abhyanga:** Self-massage with warm oil, such as sesame or almond oil, nourishes the skin, calms the mind, and improves circulation.
- **Pranayama:** Breathing exercises like alternate nostril breathing help balance energy flow and calm the mind.
- **Meditation:** Take a few minutes to center yourself and set intentions for the day ahead.

These practices help ground and prepare you for the day ahead, creating a foundation for overall well-being. Throughout the day, mindful eating practices, staying hydrated, and taking short breaks for stretching or deep breathing can further support your self-care journey.

Weekly self-care routines in Ayurveda often involve deeper rejuvenation and detoxification. Here are some examples of weekly self-care practices you can incorporate:

- **Abhyanga:** Regular self-massage with warm oil not only nourishes the skin but also supports relaxation and stress relief.

- **Soothing baths:** Adding calming essential oils like lavender or eucalyptus to your bath can help unwind and release tension.
- **Detox rituals:** Ayurvedic detox practices, such as Panchakarma, can be done seasonally to purify the body and reset your system.
- **Yoga practice:** Engaging in regular yoga practice helps balance the doshas, improves flexibility, and enhances overall well-being.
- **Nature connection:** Spending time in nature, whether it's a walk in the park or forest bathing, can recharge your energies and promote inner harmony.

Get creative with your routines - listen to uplifting music while doing your self-massage, add some humor to your meditation practice, or involve friends in a group yoga session. The key is to make self-care a pleasurable and rewarding experience that resonates with your unique personality and preferences.

Remember, self-care in Ayurveda is not a one-size-fits-all approach. It's about tuning into your body, mind, and spirit, and tailoring your practices to suit your individual needs and doshic balance. By incorporating daily and weekly self-care rituals into your routine, you'll not only enhance your overall well-being but also cultivate a deeper connection with yourself and the world around you.

Chapter 8

Mind-Body Connection

Ayurveda places great emphasis on the mind-body connection. Mental health is considered essential for maintaining balance in the body. The mind is seen as the central point where all experiences, emotions, and thoughts converge.

According to Ayurvedic principles, the mind is composed of three Gunas, or qualities: Sattva (purity, harmony), Rajas (activity, energy), and Tamas (inertia, darkness). When these Gunas are in balance, the mind is clear, focused, and stable, leading to good mental health.

However, when the mind is disturbed or imbalanced, it can lead to a disruption of the Doshas – Vata, Pitta, and Kapha). Imbalance in the Doshas can manifest as physical ailments ranging from digestive issues to chronic diseases. This highlights the intricate relationship between mental and physical health in Ayurveda.

Ayurveda views mental health holistically, considering not just the symptoms but also the root cause of any imbalance. In Ayurvedic philosophy, each individual has a unique mind-body constitution known as Prakriti, which determines their predisposition to certain mental and physical imbalances. By understanding your Prakriti, Ayurveda offers personalized recommendations for maintaining mental well-being and preventing disease.

One of the key principles in Ayurveda is the concept of Ahara (diet) and Vihara (lifestyle) as essential factors in maintaining mental health. A diet that is suitable for one's Prakriti can help balance the Doshas and promote a healthy mind. Regular exercise, meditation, and relaxation techniques are also recommended to calm the mind, reduce stress, and enhance mental clarity.

Ayurveda recognizes the mind as a powerful healer and prescribes various mental practices to maintain mental health. These practices include meditation, Pranayama (breath control), and Yoga, which are believed to have a profound impact on the mind-body system. Meditation, in particular, is considered a powerful tool for calming the mind, increasing self-awareness, and promoting emotional well-being.

Ayurveda also recognizes the influence of external factors on mental health. The environment in which we live, the people we interact with, and the activities we engage in all have an impact on our mental well-being. According to Ayurveda, creating a supportive and nurturing environment is essential for maintaining mental health. This includes surrounding oneself with positive influences, engaging in activities that bring joy and fulfillment, and cultivating meaningful relationships.

Emotional health is another aspect of mental well-being that Ayurveda places great importance on. In Ayurveda, emotions are seen as subtle energies that can influence the Doshas and, consequently, our physical health. Suppressing emotions or experiencing prolonged emotional disturbance can lead to imbalances in the Doshas and result in various health problems.

Ayurveda offers a holistic approach to mental health, addressing not just the symptoms but also the underlying causes of mental imbalances. By recognizing the interconnectedness of the mind and body, Ayurveda provides a comprehensive framework for maintaining mental well-being and preventing disease. Through a combination of diet, lifestyle modifications, mental practices, and emotional healing, Ayurveda empowers you to take charge of your mental health and lead a balanced and fulfilling life.

Meditation and Mindfulness: Techniques For Calming the Mind

At the heart of Ayurveda lies the art of mindfulness—the practice of being fully present in the here and now. In a world filled with distractions and busyness, cultivating mindfulness is like tending to the garden of your soul. It allows you to embrace each moment with awareness and intention, leading to a deep sense of contentment and inner clarity.

Meditation, the sacred art of inner contemplation, is also a powerful tool in Ayurveda for quieting the mind and nurturing the spirit. Through meditation, we learn to transcend the chatter of our thoughts and connect with the vast, silent space within us, the source of pure consciousness and infinite wisdom.

Now, let us explore some techniques and exercises to awaken your inner light and cultivate mindfulness and meditation in your daily life:

Body Scan Meditation

- Lie down in a quiet, peaceful space and close your eyes.
- Start at your toes and gradually move your awareness up through your body, noticing any sensations or areas of tension.

- As you scan each body part, gently release any tightness or discomfort, inviting relaxation and ease.

This body scan meditation promotes deep relaxation and a profound sense of connection to your physical self.

Mantra Meditation

- Choose a sacred mantra or affirmation that resonates with your heart.
- Sit in a comfortable position, close your eyes, and repeat the mantra silently or aloud.
- Let the vibration of the sacred words cleanse your mind and uplift your spirit.
- Dive deep into the ocean of your inner being, where pure love and wisdom reside.

Mindful Eating

- Before eating, take a moment to express gratitude for the nourishment before you.
- Chew each bite slowly and savor the flavors and textures.
- Be fully present with each morsel, noticing how it nourishes your body and delights your senses.

Mindful eating not only promotes digestive health but also deepens your connection to the abundance of life.

Nature Walk Meditation

- Go on a walk through a local park or natural setting, observing the intricate details of the world around you.
- Feel the earth beneath your feet, listen to the songs of birds, and inhale the fragrant scents of the forest.
- Let nature's serenity guide you into a state of profound peace and harmony.

Pranayama: Breathing Techniques for Energy and Balance

Pranayama, a Sanskrit word meaning "extension of the breath" or "extension of life force," is a key aspect of Ayurveda. The breath is seen as the vital link between the body, mind, and spirit. By controlling the breath through specific techniques, you can enhance the flow of prana, or life force, throughout your body, leading to improved health and vitality.

Now, let's delve into some breathing techniques that can help you harness the energy and balance that Pranayama has to offer:

Nadi Shodhana (Alternate Nostril Breathing)

This technique involves breathing through one nostril at a time while closing off the other nostril with your thumb. Start by inhaling through one nostril, then exhaling through the other, and continue switching back and forth.

Nadi Shodhana is known to balance the left and right hemispheres of the brain, bringing a sense of calmness and mental clarity.

Kapalabhati (Skull Shining Breath)

This dynamic breathing technique involves quick, forceful exhalations followed by passive inhalations. Kapalabhati is believed to cleanse the mind and body, increase oxygen flow, and boost energy levels.

Imagine each exhalation as a way to release any stagnant energy within you, allowing for a renewed sense of vitality.

Ujjayi (Victorious Breath)

Ujjayi breath involves breathing in and out through the nose with a slight constriction in the back of the throat, creating a soft, ocean-like sound. This technique is not only calming but also helps to build internal heat and focus the mind.

Imagine the sound of the ocean waves as you inhale and exhale, inviting a sense of peace and tranquility.

Bhramari (Bee Breath)

Bhramari involves making a humming sound while exhaling, creating a vibration that resonates throughout the body. This technique is excellent for relieving stress and anxiety and promoting deep relaxation.

Picture yourself surrounded by the gentle buzzing of bees, allowing yourself to let go of any tension and find inner peace.

Sitali (Cooling Breath)

Sitali involves rolling the tongue into a tube-like shape and inhaling through the mouth, then exhaling through the nose. This breath is cooling and soothing, making it ideal for calming the mind and reducing body heat.

Visualize a refreshing breeze flowing through your body as you practice Sitali, bringing a sense of rejuvenation and balance.

By incorporating these breathing techniques into your daily routine, you can tap into the immense benefits of Pranayama in Ayurveda. Remember, the key is to practice mindfulness and intention, allowing yourself to connect deeply with your breath and inner self.

Managing Stress and Emotions: Ayurvedic Approaches to Mental Well-being

Managing stress and emotions using Ayurvedic principles is like embarking on a journey to discover the inner harmony and peace that reside within you. Ayurveda offers a unique perspective on mental well-being by emphasizing the connection between mind, body, and spirit.

Imagine yourself as a beautiful flower swaying gently in the breeze, rooted deeply in the rich soil of your Ayurvedic wisdom. Just as flowers need sunlight, water, and care to bloom, you too can nurture your mental well-being through the practices and principles of Ayurveda.

In Ayurveda, managing stress and emotions starts with understanding your dosha. By identifying your dominant dosha, you can tailor your mental well-being practices to achieve balance and harmony.

Let's take a closer look at each dosha and the Ayurvedic approaches to managing stress and emotions:

- **Vata:** To manage stress and emotions as a Vata type, focus on grounding practices such as meditation, gentle yoga, and warm, nourishing foods. Cultivate a sense of routine and stability to calm your busy mind and soothe your spirit.
- **Pitta:** To support your mental well-being as a Pitta type, practice cooling and calming activities like swimming, spending time in nature, and engaging in creative expression. Avoid situations that trigger your competitiveness, and learn to let go of control to find inner peace.

- **Kapha:** To maintain mental well-being as a Kapha type, engage in energizing activities like hiking, dancing, and practicing invigorating pranayama (breathwork). Cultivate a sense of lightness and playfulness to uplift your spirit and dispel any stagnant energy.

In addition to understanding your dosha, Ayurveda offers a variety of holistic practices to support your mental well-being:

- **Abhyanga:** Take time each day to massage your limbs in gentle, circular motions, allowing the healing properties of the oils to penetrate your skin and calm your nervous system.

- **Pranayama:** Practice deep, mindful breathing exercises such as Nadi Shodhana (alternate nostril breathing) or Bhramari (humming bee breath) to clear your mind, balance your energy, and promote relaxation.

- **Sattvic Diet:** Ayurveda emphasizes the importance of eating sattvic foods - fresh, organic, and minimally processed to nourish your body and mind. Include a variety of fruits, vegetables, whole grains, and healthy fats in your diet to maintain mental clarity, digestive health, and emotional balance.

- **Mindfulness and Meditation:** Cultivate mindfulness through practices such as meditation, yoga, or simply taking moments throughout the day to pause, breathe, and connect with the present moment. By being fully present and aware, you can cultivate inner peace and resilience in the face of stress and emotional challenges.

- **Nature Connection:** Spending time in nature is a powerful way to rejuvenate your mind, body, and spirit. Take walks in the forest, sit by a tranquil lake, or simply bask in the warmth of the sun to reconnect with the natural rhythms of life and find inner tranquility.

Chapter 9

An Ayurvedic Approach to Exercise

We know that in Ayurveda, keeping the body in balance is of utmost importance, and exercise plays a key role in achieving and maintaining that balance. When you move your body through exercise, you're not only strengthening your muscles and improving your cardiovascular health, but you're also boosting your metabolism, improving digestion, and helping to release toxins from your system.

From an Ayurvedic perspective, engaging in the right type and amount of exercise can help bring all three doshas back into harmony. For example, if you're feeling sluggish and heavy, invigorating activities like brisk walking or yoga can help stimulate your energy and uplift your mood. On the other hand, if you're feeling anxious or overheated, cooling exercises like swimming or gentle stretching can help calm your mind and soothe your body.

So, whether you're into yoga, dancing, hiking, or even just going for a leisurely stroll in nature, remember that each movement you make is a step towards better health and well-being in the eyes of Ayurveda.

Exercise and Doshas: Finding the Right Type of Exercise for Your Dosha

When it comes to choosing the right type of exercise for your dosha, Ayurveda offers insightful guidance tailored to individual needs. Let's explore how you can align your workout routine with your dosha to optimize your health and vitality.

Vata Dosha

If your constitution is predominantly Vata, characterized by qualities of air and space, you may benefit from grounding, nurturing, and calming exercises. Vata types are prone to being light, quick-witted, and creative but can also experience tendencies towards anxiety and instability.

To balance Vata dosha, opt for exercises that provide stability and grounding, such as yoga, Tai Chi, or gentle strength training. These activities can help calm the restless energy of Vata and promote a sense of centeredness and focus. Engaging in regular, rhythmic movements can also support Vata types in establishing a sense of routine and stability.

Pitta Dosha

If you have a dominant Pitta dosha embodies qualities of fire and water, exhibiting traits of ambition, intensity, and sharp intellect. Pitta types are prone to heat-related imbalances, such as inflammation and irritability, and can benefit from cooling and soothing forms of exercise.

For Pitta dosha, activities that promote balance, relaxation, and a sense of flow are ideal. Swimming, cycling, or Pilates are excellent choices for Pitta types, as they offer a combination of physical challenge and mental focus without excessive intensity. These workouts can help Pitta individuals channel their competitive drive in healthy ways and prevent overheating or burnout.

Kapha Dosha

Kapha dosha, embodying the qualities of earth and water, is characterized by stability, endurance, and nurturing tendencies. Kapha types often have strong, sturdy physiques but can struggle with sluggishness, lethargy, and weight gain if imbalanced.

To balance Kapha dosha, opt for energizing, invigorating exercises that promote movement and circulation. High-intensity interval training (HIIT), dancing, or hiking are excellent choices for Kapha types, as they help stimulate metabolism, build strength, and uplift the spirits. These dynamic workouts can help Kapha individuals combat stagnation and enhance their vitality and motivation.

While aligning your exercise routine with your dosha can be beneficial, it's important to remember that we're all unique, and a holistic approach to health considers individual variations beyond doshic influences. Listen to your body's cues, observe how different types of exercise make you feel, and adjust your workout regimen accordingly.

Incorporating mindfulness practices such as deep breathing, meditation, or self-reflection can also enhance the benefits of exercise and support overall doshic balance. Remember to stay hydrated, eat nourishing foods aligned with your dosha, and prioritize rest and recovery to complement your physical activities.

Yoga and Ayurveda: The Synergy Between Yoga and Ayurvedic Practices

Yoga and Ayurveda are two ancient practices that have been intertwined for centuries, offering a synergistic approach to health and wellness.

Yoga, originating from ancient India, is a practice that combines physical postures (asanas), breathing techniques (pranayama), meditation, and philosophy to promote overall well-being.

The synergy between Yoga and Ayurveda lies in their shared emphasis on self-awareness, balance, and harmony. Both practices recognize the interconnectedness of the body, mind, and spirit, viewing health as a holistic experience that encompasses all aspects of one's being.

We know that in Ayurveda, each person is believed to possess a unique mind-body constitution, known as doshas, which influence their physical and emotional tendencies. Similarly, Yoga recognizes the importance of individualized practices, encouraging us to listen to our bodies and honor our personal limits.

Yoga Asanas for Each Dosha

- **Vata Dosha:** Grounding poses such as Warrior I, Tree Pose, and Child's Pose help to calm an overactive Vata energy, reducing anxiety and improving focus.
- **Pitta Dosha:** Cooling poses like the Extended Triangle Pose, Forward Fold, and Cobra Pose are beneficial for balancing Pitta dosha, releasing tension, and promoting relaxation.
- **Kapha Dosha:** Invigorating poses such as Bridge Pose, Half Moon Pose, and Camel Pose can stimulate Kapha energy, boosting metabolism and uplifting mood.

Ayurvedic Self-Massage (Abhyanga)

Before or after your Yoga practice, indulge in a nourishing self-massage using warm sesame or coconut oil. This Ayurvedic practice helps to promote circulation, relax the muscles, and balance the doshas, leaving you feeling rejuvenated and centered.

Meditation and Mindfulness

Conclude your practice with a few minutes of meditation or mindfulness to cultivate inner peace, clarity, and spiritual connection. Focus on your breath, observe your thoughts without judgment, and cultivate a sense of gratitude for the present moment.

As you explore the connection between Yoga and Ayurveda, remember to approach your practice with curiosity, compassion, and a sense of playfulness. Allow yourself to experiment with different techniques, listen to your body's needs, and honor your unique journey towards holistic well-being.

By integrating the wisdom of Yoga and Ayurveda into your daily life, you can create a harmonious balance between body, mind, and spirit, nurturing optimal health and vitality.

Creating an Exercise Routine: Tips for a Balanced and Sustainable Practice

When it comes to designing an exercise routine that aligns with Ayurvedic principles, there are a few key factors to consider to ensure that you are nurturing yourself in a holistic way.

We've already covered the importance of identifying your dominant dosha and choosing exercises that align with it.

It is also important to consider the time of day when you choose to exercise, as Ayurveda places great emphasis on the cyclic nature of the body's energies. According to Ayurvedic principles, the best time to engage in physical activity is during the Kapha time of day, which is from 6 am to 10 am. This is when your energy and strength are naturally at their peak, making it easier to enjoy your workout and reap its benefits.

In addition to choosing the right type of exercise and the optimal time of day, it is essential to listen to your body and practice mindfulness during your workouts. Pay attention to how your body responds to different movements and adjust your routine accordingly. If you feel fatigued or experience pain, it may be a sign that you need to dial back the intensity or switch to a different form of exercise.

Another key aspect of creating a balanced and sustainable exercise routine in Ayurveda is incorporating self-care practices to support your body's recovery and rejuvenation. This could include activities like Abhyanga (self-massage with warm oil), Shirodhara (oil pouring on the forehead), or Pranayama (breathwork) to help calm the mind and nurture your body after a workout.

Lastly, remember that consistency is key when it comes to maintaining a healthy exercise routine. Instead of pushing yourself to the limit with sporadic intense workouts, aim for regular, moderate exercise that you enjoy and can sustain in the long run. This will not only help you stay motivated but also prevent burnout and injury. Remember, you don't have to join the gym and go every single day; you simply need to find a routine that you enjoy and that brings you benefits.

Recovery and Rest: Importance of Rest in Maintaining Health

Rest and recovery are fundamental aspects of Ayurveda. Maintaining a balance between activity and rest is considered essential for overall well-being and optimal health. Just as a plant needs time to rest and rejuvenate to flourish, so too do our bodies and minds require periods of rest to replenish and restore their vital energies.

At the heart of Ayurvedic philosophy lies the concept of balance, known as "Sattva." This balance encompasses not only our physical state but also our mental and emotional well-being. Proper rest and recovery play a pivotal role in maintaining this delicate equilibrium. When we push ourselves beyond our limits, ignoring the signs of fatigue and burnout, we disrupt the natural rhythm of our bodies and minds, setting the stage for imbalances and dis-ease.

So, how can you ensure that you prioritize rest and recovery in your daily life, in alignment with Ayurvedic principles? Here are some tips to help you infuse your routine with a little rest:

- **Listen to your body:** Your body is a wise and intuitive guide, always communicating its needs to you. Pay attention to signals of fatigue, such as low energy, irritability, or difficulty concentrating. When your body whispers, "I need rest," listen attentively and honor its request.
- **Establish a bedtime routine:** Ayurveda emphasizes the importance of aligning our daily routine with the natural rhythms of the day. Set a regular bedtime and create a calming bedtime ritual to signal to your body that it's time to wind down. This could include activities like gentle stretching, reading a book, or practicing relaxation techniques like meditation or deep breathing.

- **Unplug and unwind:** In our hyper-connected world, it's easy to be constantly plugged into technology, and bombarded by notifications and stimuli. Make a conscious effort to unplug at least an hour before bedtime to allow your mind to unwind and prepare for restful sleep.

- **Nourish your body with restorative practices:** Ayurveda offers a treasure trove of restorative practices to replenish your energy reserves. Try incorporating practices like Abhyanga (self-massage with warm oil), Shirodhara (pouring warm oil on the forehead), or Nidra Yoga (yogic sleep) into your routine to promote deep relaxation and rejuvenation.

- **Simplify your schedule:** In the pursuit of productivity and achievement, we often overload our schedules with commitments and activities. Simplify your schedule by prioritizing your tasks, learning to say no when necessary, and creating space for rest and leisure. Remember, productivity is not just about doing more; it's about doing what truly matters.

- **Connect with nature:** Spending time in nature is a potent elixir for the body and soul. Take a leisurely stroll in a park, breathe in the fresh air, or simply sit and soak in the sights and sounds of your natural surroundings. Nature has a calming and grounding effect, helping you disconnect from the chaos of everyday life and reconnect with your inner peace.

- **Practice mindfulness:** Mindfulness is the art of being fully present in the moment, without judgment or distraction. Cultivate mindfulness in your daily activities, whether it's eating a meal, washing dishes, or going for a walk. By immersing yourself in the present moment, you can experience a sense of calm and relaxation that transcends external stressors.

- **Seek professional guidance:** If you're struggling to prioritize rest and recovery or experiencing chronic fatigue, consider seeking guidance from an Ayurvedic practitioner or holistic health coach. They can provide personalized recommendations tailored to your unique constitution and health needs, helping you navigate the path to optimal well-being.

In the end, rest and recovery are not luxuries but vital components of a balanced and vibrant life. By honoring the wisdom of Ayurveda and embracing the art of rest, you can cultivate a deeper sense of harmony, vitality, and joy in your journey towards holistic wellness.

Chapter 10

Ayurveda and Disease Prevention

Ayurveda is like that wise old friend who always reminds you to take care of yourself before things go haywire. Imagine a world where you could avoid getting sick by simply aligning your lifestyle with the rhythms of nature. That's what Ayurveda is all about.

Preventative health in Ayurveda starts with understanding your own doshic constitution and making choices that support it. By following a lifestyle that aligns with your dominant dosha, you can maintain balance and ward off illness before it even stands a chance. For example, if you are predominantly Vata, focusing on grounding activities, warm, nourishing foods, and regular routines can help keep your mind and body in equilibrium.

But it's not just about what you eat or how you move your body – Ayurveda also emphasizes the importance of mental and emotional well-being in preventing illness.

Stress, anxiety, and negative emotions can disrupt the doshic balance and weaken your immune system, making you more susceptible to disease. That's why practices like meditation, yoga, and pranayama (breathwork) are vital components of an Ayurvedic lifestyle, helping to calm the mind, reduce stress, and promote overall well-being.

Another key aspect of preventative health in Ayurveda is the concept of seasonal routines. Just like nature goes through its own cycles, our bodies also respond to the changing seasons. By adapting our diet, exercise, and self-care practices according to the time of year, we can support our body's natural ability to stay healthy and resilient. For example, in the cold winter months, focusing on warming foods and staying hydrated can help balance the Vata dosha and prevent common winter ailments like colds and flu.

Ayurveda also places a strong emphasis on daily routines, known as dinacharya, which help to establish a sense of structure and stability in your life. From waking up with the sun to practicing oil pulling and tongue scraping, these simple yet powerful rituals can have a profound impact on your overall health and well-being. By incorporating these practices into your daily routine, you create a solid foundation for preventative health and set yourself up for long-term wellness.

In addition to lifestyle practices, Ayurveda also offers a wide range of herbal remedies, dietary supplements, and therapies to support the body's natural healing abilities and prevent illness. From rejuvenating tonics like Ashwagandha and Triphala to detoxifying treatments like Panchakarma, Ayurveda provides a holistic approach to health that addresses the root cause of imbalances rather than just masking symptoms.

But perhaps the most powerful aspect of Ayurveda's preventative health approach is its emphasis on self-awareness and self-care. By tuning into your body's signals and heeding its wisdom, you can make informed choices that support your health and well-being. Whether it's taking time to rest when you feel tired, nourishing yourself with wholesome foods, or engaging in practices that bring you joy and relaxation, Ayurveda teaches us to listen to our bodies and take proactive steps to prevent illness before it takes hold.

So, the next time you feel tempted to push through fatigue, ignore stress or indulge in unhealthy habits, remember the wisdom of Ayurveda that true health is not just the absence of disease but a vibrant state of balance and harmony that comes from taking care of yourself on all levels.

Strengthening Immunity: Ayurvedic Practices for a Robust Immune System

Ayurveda views immunity as the body's ability to defend against disease-causing agents and maintain balance. According to Ayurvedic principles, a robust immune system is closely linked to the balance of the three doshas and the optimal functioning of the body's digestive fire, or Agni.

Agni in Ayurveda refers to the digestive fire or digestive power within the body. It is responsible for the digestion, absorption, and assimilation of food, as well as the transformation of food into energy. A balanced Agni is essential for overall health and well-being, according to Ayurvedic principles.

If Agni is weak or imbalanced, it can lead to various health issues, such as indigestion, bloating, and decreased immunity. Ayurveda focuses on maintaining and strengthening Agni through proper diet, lifestyle practices, and herbal remedies to support optimal digestion and overall health.

When the doshas are in harmony and Agni is strong, the body is better equipped to fight off pathogens and maintain health.

Ayurvedic Practices to Strengthen Immunity

- **Balance Your Doshas:** To enhance immunity, it's essential to balance the doshas through diet, lifestyle, and herbal remedies. Determine your unique doshic constitution and incorporate foods and practices that support equilibrium. For example, Vata types may benefit from warming and grounding foods; Pitta individuals can focus on cooling and soothing choices; and Kapha individuals should opt for light and stimulating options.

- **Support Digestive Fire:** Ayurveda places great importance on maintaining a healthy digestive system for strong immunity. To strengthen Agni, consume warm and cooked foods, avoid overeating, and incorporate digestive spices like ginger, cumin, and turmeric into your meals. Additionally, practicing mindful eating and avoiding processed foods can aid in improving digestion and the assimilation of nutrients.

- **Herbal Support:** Ayurveda offers a plethora of herbs known for their immune-boosting properties. Some popular choices include Ashwagandha, Tulsi (Holy Basil), Amalaki (Indian Gooseberry), and Triphala. These herbs not only strengthen the immune system but also promote overall well-being and vitality. Incorporate these herbs into your daily routine through teas, supplements, or Ayurvedic formulations.

- **Daily Routine:** Establishing a daily routine, or Dinacharya, is crucial for maintaining balance and supporting immunity. Wake up early, practice self-care rituals like oil massage (Abhyanga) and tongue scraping, engage in regular exercise or yoga and prioritize restorative sleep. Consistency in daily habits plays a significant role in enhancing overall health and immunity.

- **Stress Management:** Chronic stress can weaken the immune system and disrupt the body's natural defenses. Ayurveda emphasizes the importance of managing stress through practices like meditation, pranayama (breathwork), and mindfulness. Incorporate stress-relieving techniques into your routine to promote emotional well-being and immunity.

- **Detoxification:** Toxins, or Ama, accumulate in the body due to poor digestion and lifestyle choices, compromising immunity. Ayurveda recommends periodic detoxification practices, such as Panchakarma therapy, to eliminate Ama and rejuvenate the body. Consult with an Ayurvedic practitioner to determine the most suitable detox plan for your individual needs.

- **Seasonal Adaptation:** Ayurveda recognizes the influence of seasonal changes on health and immunity. Adjust your diet and lifestyle habits according to the seasons to align with nature's rhythms and prevent imbalances. For example, favor warm and nourishing foods in the winter and light and hydrating foods in the summer to support your immune system during different seasons.

- **Hydration and Nourishment:** Stay hydrated and nourished to support your immune system. Drink warm water throughout the day and consume hydrating foods like soups, stews, and herbal teas. Opt for organic, fresh, and seasonal produce to provide your body with essential nutrients and antioxidants.

Start by assessing your current lifestyle habits and identifying areas where you can introduce Ayurvedic principles. Remember, consistency is key when it comes to reaping the benefits of these time-honored practices.

You could also create a personalized wellness plan incorporating Ayurvedic dietary recommendations, herbal supplements, stress-relief techniques, and daily rituals. If it helps, consult with an Ayurvedic practitioner for tailored guidance and support in implementing these practices effectively.

Understanding Disease in Ayurveda: Causes and Progression of Diseases

In Ayurveda, the onset of disease is seen as a gradual process that begins with the accumulation of toxins and imbalances in the body. These imbalances can be caused by a variety of factors, including poor diet, lack of exercise, stress, and environmental toxins.

Let's imagine a scenario where someone follows an unhealthy diet that is high in processed foods, sugar, and fats. Over time, this person's digestive system becomes compromised, leading to a buildup of toxins and impurities in the body. As a result, their Pitta dosha becomes out of balance, causing inflammation, indigestion, and skin problems.

If left unaddressed, this imbalance could eventually lead to the progression of more serious diseases, such as diabetes, heart disease, or autoimmune disorders. Ayurveda teaches us that by understanding the root causes of these imbalances and making changes to our lifestyle and habits, we can prevent the progression of disease and promote overall health and well-being.

By paying attention to the early signs of imbalance in the body, such as fatigue, digestive issues, or skin problems, we can address these issues before they progress into more serious health problems. Ayurveda teaches us to listen to our bodies, trust our intuition, and make choices that support our unique constitution and doshic balance.

Let's explore some of the diseases and conditions that Ayurveda commonly addresses:

- **Digestive Disorders:** Ayurveda places great emphasis on digestion, considering it a cornerstone of health. Conditions like indigestion, bloating, Irritable Bowel Syndrome (IBS), and acid reflux are often attributed to imbalances in the digestive fire, known as Agni. Ayurvedic treatments aim to strengthen Agni through dietary modifications, herbal remedies, and lifestyle changes.

- **Stress and Anxiety:** In our fast-paced modern world, stress and anxiety have become all too common. Ayurveda views these conditions as imbalances in the nervous system and mental well-being. Practices such as meditation, yoga, and Ayurvedic herbs like Ashwagandha are recommended to calm the mind and restore balance.

- **Skin Disorders:** Conditions like eczema, psoriasis, and acne are often associated with imbalances in the Pitta dosha, which governs digestion and metabolism. Ayurvedic treatments focus on reducing inflammation, purifying the blood, and promoting skin health through a proper diet, herbal remedies, and detoxification therapies.

- **Respiratory Issues:** Asthma, bronchitis, and allergies can be linked to imbalances in the Kapha dosha, which governs mucous and fluid balance in the body. Ayurvedic treatments aim to clear excess mucous, strengthen the respiratory system, and boost immunity through herbal formulas, steam therapy, and breathing exercises.
- **Joint Pain and Arthritis:** Conditions like osteoarthritis and rheumatoid arthritis are often attributed to imbalances in the Vata dosha, which governs movement and nerve impulses. Ayurvedic treatments focus on reducing inflammation, lubricating joints, and improving circulation through diet, lifestyle adjustments, and herbal remedies like turmeric and ginger.
- **Hormonal Imbalance:** Disorders like PCOS, endometriosis, and thyroid imbalances are often related to disruptions in hormonal levels. Ayurveda addresses these imbalances by focusing on diet, stress management, and herbal supplements to support hormonal equilibrium and overall well-being.
- **Heart Health:** Ayurveda recognizes the importance of maintaining a healthy heart to promote longevity and vitality. Conditions like high blood pressure, cholesterol imbalances, and heart disease are approached through diet, lifestyle changes, and

herbal remedies that support heart health and circulation.

As you can see, Ayurveda offers a comprehensive approach to treating a wide range of diseases and conditions by addressing the root causes of imbalances in the body and mind. By restoring harmony to the doshas through personalized treatments and lifestyle modifications, Ayurveda aims to not only alleviate symptoms but also promote long-lasting health and wellness.

Common Ailments and Remedies: Ayurvedic Solutions for Everyday Issues.

To show you just how useful and flexible Ayurveda is, let's explore common ailments that we all face in our everyday lives and discover some Ayurvedic remedies to help alleviate these issues.

- **Digestive Issues:** One of the most common complaints we hear about is digestive issues. From bloating and indigestion to constipation and gas, our digestive system can get a bit out of whack sometimes. One Ayurvedic remedy for improving digestion is to drink a warm glass of water with freshly squeezed lemon juice first thing in the morning. This helps kick-start your digestive system and detoxify your body.

- **Stress and Anxiety:** In today's fast-paced world, stress and anxiety seem to be constant companions for many of us. Ayurveda recommends incorporating daily meditation and mindfulness practices to help calm the mind and reduce stress levels. Additionally, drinking calming herbal teas like chamomile or ashwagandha can also help alleviate anxiety symptoms.

- **Common Cold and Flu:** During the colder months, it's not uncommon to come down with a cold or the flu. Ayurveda suggests boosting your immune system with the use of spices like turmeric, ginger, and garlic in your cooking. You can also try steam inhalation with eucalyptus oil to help clear out congestion and ease breathing.

- **Insomnia:** For those nights when sleep just won't come, Ayurveda offers various remedies to promote a restful night's sleep. Try drinking a warm cup of golden milk (milk mixed with turmeric and other spices) before bedtime to help relax your body and mind. You can also practice gentle yoga poses or try a soothing lavender essential oil diffuser to create a calming atmosphere.

- **Headaches:** Whether it's tension headaches from stress or migraines triggered by various factors, Ayurveda has some solutions to offer. Rubbing a few drops of peppermint oil on your temples can help alleviate headache symptoms. Massaging your scalp with warm sesame oil can also help relax tense muscles and improve circulation.

- **Skin Issues:** From acne and eczema to dry skin and wrinkles, our skin can sometimes be a source of frustration. Ayurveda recommends incorporating a daily skincare routine using natural ingredients like neem, turmeric, and aloe vera to address various skin concerns. Drinking plenty of water and consuming foods rich in antioxidants can also help promote healthy, glowing skin.

- **Menstrual Cramps:** For those days when menstrual cramps make it hard to function, Ayurveda offers some remedies to ease the pain. Drinking warm herbal teas like ginger or cinnamon can help soothe cramps and improve blood circulation. Applying a warm compress to your lower abdomen or practicing gentle yoga poses can also provide relief.

- **Allergies:** Seasonal allergies can be a real nuisance for many people. Ayurveda suggests incorporating immune-boosting foods like honey, turmeric, and local raw honey into your diet to help reduce allergy symptoms. Using a neti pot with saline solution can also help clear out nasal passages and relieve congestion.

By incorporating these Ayurvedic remedies into your daily routine, you can help support your body's natural healing processes and achieve overall well-being.

Chapter 11

Ayurveda Across the Lifespan

The wisdom of Ayurveda can enrich and support every stage of life with its time-tested principles. From infancy to old age, Ayurveda offers a treasure trove of knowledge to enhance well-being and vitality.

Imagine each chapter of life as a unique canvas, waiting to be painted with the vibrant colors of Ayurvedic practices. Just as a skilled artist brings depth and beauty to a masterpiece, Ayurveda guides us to harmonize our body, mind, and spirit in perfect alignment with the rhythms of nature.

Ayurvedic Practices for Different Life Stages: Childhood, Adulthood, and Old Age

Let's take a look at some Ayurvedic practices for different life stages: childhood, adulthood, and old age, with a little actionable advice thrown in for good measure.

Childhood: Planting the Seeds for Health and Well-being

In the tender years of childhood, the foundation for lifelong health is laid. Ayurveda emphasizes the importance of balance and nurturing during this critical stage.

Here are some Ayurvedic practices for promoting well-being in children:

- **Balanced Nutrition:** Understanding your child's dosha can help tailor their diet to maintain balance. Aim for a diet rich in whole foods, organic fruits, vegetables, and grains to nourish their growing bodies.

- **Daily Routine:** Establishing a daily routine for children creates a sense of stability and promotes good health. Encourage regular meal times, and proper sleep, and balance their activities with play and rest. Incorporate fun activities like yoga and meditation to foster mindfulness and a connection to their inner selves.

- **Herbal Support:** Herbal remedies can be beneficial for children to support their immune system, digestion, and overall well-being. Consult with an Ayurvedic practitioner to choose safe and effective herbs for your child's specific needs.

- **Emotional Well-being:** Emotional health is paramount in childhood development. Encourage open communication, provide a loving and nurturing environment, and teach them coping mechanisms such as deep breathing exercises or journaling to deal with stress and emotions.

Adulthood: Nurturing the Fire of Life

As we transition into adulthood, the focus shifts to balancing responsibilities, careers, relationships, and self-care. Ayurvedic principles offer guidance on maintaining vitality and harmony during this stage:

- **Diet and Digestion:** The digestive fire, Agni, plays a crucial role in overall health. Incorporate warm, cooked foods, spices like ginger and turmeric, and herbal teas to support digestion. Avoid processed foods, excessive caffeine, and alcohol, which can dampen Agni.

- **Stress Management:** The demands of adulthood can lead to increased stress levels. Practice mindfulness, meditation, and yoga to manage stress effectively. Engage in grounding activities like spending time in nature, listening to soothing music, or indulging in self-care rituals to nurture your mind and body.

- **Physical Activity:** Regular exercise is vital for maintaining physical health and balancing doshas. Choose activities that align with your body type and preferences, whether it's yoga, strength training, or dancing. Listen to your body's cues and adjust your routine accordingly.

- **Sleep Hygiene:** Quality sleep is essential for rejuvenation and overall well-being. Establish a calming bedtime routine, create a peaceful sleep environment, and wind down with relaxing activities before bed. Aim for 7-9 hours of restful sleep each night to support optimal health.

Old Age: Embracing Wisdom and Grace

In the golden years of old age, Ayurveda emphasizes the importance of preserving vitality, wisdom, and adaptability. Here are some actionable practices to promote wellness in old age:

- **Mind-Body Connection:** Maintain a strong connection between mind and body through practices such as meditation, pranayama (breathwork), and gentle yoga. These practices can help enhance mental clarity, emotional balance, and physical agility.
- **Nutritious Diet:** As we age, our nutritional needs may change. Focus on nourishing, easily digestible foods such as cooked vegetables, whole grains, and plant-based proteins. Include herbs and spices like ashwagandha, turmeric, and tulsi to support vitality and immunity.

- **Joint Health:** Joint stiffness and mobility issues are common in old age. Incorporate gentle exercises, such as Tai Chi or water aerobics, to maintain joint flexibility and strength. Consider Ayurvedic remedies like massage with warm oils or herbal supplements for joint support.

- **Community and Connection:** Stay socially engaged and maintain relationships with loved ones to foster a sense of belonging and purpose. Participate in community activities, volunteer work, or pursue hobbies and interests that bring joy and fulfillment.

As you can see, Ayurveda offers a holistic approach to health and well-being that transcends age boundaries. By incorporating Ayurvedic practices tailored to each life stage, you can cultivate balance, vitality, and harmony in body, mind, and spirit. Remember, wellness is a journey, and embracing the wisdom of Ayurveda can guide you towards a life of thriving in every season.

Pregnancy and Postpartum Care: Special Considerations for Mothers

In Ayurveda, pregnancy is viewed as a sacred time when the mother's body undergoes significant changes to nurture and support the growing life within her. It's essential to focus on balancing the doshas, especially Vata, during this delicate period. The good news is that Ayurveda has plenty of help for mothers and mothers-to-be.

To support the mother's health during pregnancy, Ayurveda recommends a nourishing diet rich in warm, cooked foods that are easy to digest. Incorporating foods like ghee, cooked vegetables, grains, and herbal teas can help to maintain balance and provide essential nutrients for both mother and baby.

Ayurvedic practitioners also recommend gentle forms of exercise, such as prenatal yoga and daily walks, to keep the body strong and flexible. Rest and relaxation are equally important, as stress can have a negative impact on the mother's and baby's well-being.

After childbirth, the mother enters the postpartum period, where her body undergoes a process of recovery and rejuvenation. Ayurveda places great emphasis on postpartum care to support the mother in restoring her strength and vitality.

One of the key practices in postpartum care is the use of Ayurvedic oils for self-massage, known as Abhyanga. This gentle massage helps to nourish the skin, improve circulation, and promote relaxation. Warm oil infused with herbs like ashwagandha and bala can be particularly beneficial for new mothers.

Ayurvedic dietary recommendations during the postpartum period focus on warming, nourishing foods that are easy to digest. Foods like Kitchari, a traditional Ayurvedic dish made with rice, mung beans, and warming spices, are often recommended to support the mother's recovery and promote healing.

Emotional and Spiritual Support

Ayurveda recognizes the importance of emotional and spiritual well-being during pregnancy and postpartum. Practices like meditation, pranayama (breathing exercises), and mindfulness can help mothers cultivate mental clarity, emotional balance, and spiritual connection during this transformative time.

It's essential for mothers to prioritize self-care and seek support from loved ones, healthcare providers, and Ayurvedic practitioners. Creating a nurturing and supportive environment can greatly enhance the mother's experience and promote a smooth transition into motherhood.

Aging Gracefully: Ayurvedic Strategies for Healthy Aging

Unfortunately, old age is something that comes to us all. Nobody has found the fountain of youth yet! So, while aging is a natural process that we all go through, how we age is within our control.

In Ayurveda, there are time-tested strategies for aging gracefully and maintaining optimal health and vitality. Let's explore how you can incorporate Ayurvedic principles into your life to support healthy aging.

First and foremost, Ayurveda emphasizes the importance of balance in all aspects of life – physical, mental, and emotional. As we age, it becomes even more crucial to pay attention to maintaining this balance to support our overall well-being. By understanding your dosha and incorporating foods that are suitable for your constitution, you can support healthy aging and prevent imbalances.

For example, if you have a Vata constitution, which is associated with qualities such as dryness and coldness, you may benefit from incorporating warm, nourishing foods like cooked grains, root vegetables, and warming spices into your diet. On the other hand, if you have a Pitta constitution, characterized by qualities like heat and intensity, you may benefit from cooling foods like fresh fruits, vegetables, and herbs. By aligning your diet with your dosha, you can support your body's natural balance and promote healthy aging.

In addition to diet, Ayurveda emphasizes the importance of regular physical activity to maintain strength, flexibility, and vitality as we age. Practices like yoga and meditation are highly recommended for supporting overall well-being and promoting longevity. Yoga not only helps to strengthen the body but also calms the mind and reduces stress, which is crucial for healthy aging. Even simple practices like walking in nature or gentle stretching exercises can have profound benefits for your physical and mental health.

Furthermore, Ayurveda places great importance on the concept of Ojas. In Ayurveda, Ojas refers to the vital essence of the body, which governs immunity, strength, and overall vitality. It is considered the foundation of good health and well-being.

Ojas is said to be the final byproduct of digestion and is responsible for nourishing all the tissues of the body. It is also believed to be the subtle essence of all bodily tissues and provides resilience against disease. Maintaining and nourishing Ojas is essential for optimal health, according to Ayurvedic principles.

So, as we age, it's essential to nourish and support our Ojas to maintain optimal health and vitality. One way to do this is by incorporating adaptogenic herbs like Ashwagandha, Shatavari, and Tulsi into your routine. These herbs are known for their rejuvenating and immune-boosting properties and can help support your body's resilience to stress and illness.

Another key aspect of aging gracefully in Ayurveda is maintaining a healthy digestive system. According to

Ayurveda, strong digestion is the cornerstone of good health, and poor digestion can lead to a variety of health issues as we age. To support your digestion, it's essential to eat mindfully, chew your food thoroughly, and avoid overeating. Additionally, incorporating digestive spices like ginger, cumin, and fennel into your meals can help stimulate digestion and prevent digestive issues.

In Ayurveda, daily routines, or Dinacharya are highly recommended for promoting health and longevity. Establishing a daily routine that includes practices like oil pulling, self-massage with warm oil, and meditation can help balance your doshas, calm your mind, and support healthy aging. Oil pulling, in particular, is a traditional Ayurvedic practice that involves swishing oil in your mouth to improve oral health, support detoxification, and promote overall well-being.

Furthermore, Ayurveda emphasizes the importance of rest and relaxation for healthy aging. Getting an adequate amount of quality sleep is crucial for rejuvenating the body and mind, supporting immune function, and maintaining optimal health. In Ayurveda, it is recommended to go to bed early and wake up with the sunrise to align with the body's natural rhythms. Creating a calming bedtime routine, such as sipping herbal tea, practicing relaxation techniques, or reading a book, can help promote restful sleep and support healthy aging.

Lastly, maintaining strong social connections and a sense of purpose are essential aspects of aging gracefully in Ayurveda. Building meaningful relationships, engaging in activities that bring you joy, and cultivating a sense of gratitude can have a profound impact on your overall well-being as you age. Connecting with loved ones, volunteering in your community, or pursuing hobbies and interests that light you up can help you stay vibrant and engaged in life.

Adapting Practices Over Time: How to Evolve Your Routine With Age

As we journey through life, our bodies and needs change, and it's important to adapt our Ayurvedic practices to suit our evolving selves. Let's take a look at how to evolve your Ayurvedic routine with age so you can continue to support your health and vitality at every stage of life.

In your 20s: Lay the Foundation

Your 20s are a time of youthful energy and vitality, but it's also a crucial period for establishing healthy habits that will support you in the years to come. In Ayurveda, this is the Kapha stage of life, where energy and growth are at their peak. It's important to focus on establishing a daily routine that nurtures your mind, body, and spirit.

Start your day with a gentle yoga practice or meditation to center yourself and set a positive tone for the day ahead. Incorporate plenty of fresh, seasonal fruits and vegetables into your diet to provide your body with essential nutrients and support digestion. Stay hydrated by drinking plenty of water and herbal teas throughout the day.

As you navigate the demands of work, relationships, and social life, be mindful of your stress levels and make time for self-care activities that help you relax and recharge. This can be as simple as taking a leisurely walk in nature, indulging in a warm bath with calming essential oils or practicing deep breathing exercises to calm the mind.

In your 30s: Focus on Balance

In your 30s, you may find yourself juggling the responsibilities of a career, family, and personal growth. This is the Pitta stage of life in Ayurveda, characterized by focus, ambition, and drive. It's important to focus on maintaining balance in all areas of your life to prevent burnout and support your overall well-being.

Make self-care a priority by carving out time each day for activities that help you relax and recharge. This could be a restorative yoga practice, a leisurely walk in the park, or a relaxing cup of herbal tea before bed. Pay attention to your diet and make sure to include foods that support digestion and help manage stress, such as whole grains, leafy greens, and calming herbal teas.

Incorporate Ayurvedic practices such as self-massage with warm oil (abhyanga) to nourish your skin, calm your nervous system, and promote relaxation. Practice mindfulness and be present in the moment, whether you're enjoying a meal with loved ones, taking a walk in nature, or simply sitting quietly and observing your thoughts.

In your 40s: Embrace Change

As you enter your 40s, you may notice shifts in your body and energy levels that require adjustments to your Ayurvedic routine. This is the Vata stage of life, characterized by movement, change, and creativity. It's important to embrace these changes and adapt your practices to suit your evolving needs.

Focus on incorporating grounding practices into your daily routine, such as yoga poses that help you feel centered and rooted or meditation techniques that help calm a busy mind. Pay attention to your diet and include nourishing, warming foods that support digestion and help balance Vata energy, such as soups, stews, and cooked grains.

Prioritize self-care activities that help you feel grounded and connected to yourself, such as spending time in nature, journaling, or practicing deep breathing exercises. Make time for regular exercise that helps you stay active and energized, whether it's a daily walk, a yoga class, or a dance session in your living room.

In your 50s and beyond: Cultivate Wisdom

As you move into your 50s and beyond, you have the opportunity to cultivate wisdom and embrace the fullness of life experience. This is a time to reflect on your journey, honor your body's needs, and embrace practices that support your health and vitality as you age gracefully.

Focus on gentle, restorative practices that nourish your body and spirit, such as restorative yoga, gentle stretching, or meditation. Pay attention to your diet and include foods that support digestion and nourish your body, such as warm soups, cooked vegetables, and herbal teas.

Prioritize self-care activities that help you feel grounded and present, such as spending time with loved ones, engaging in creative pursuits, or practicing gratitude. Embrace Ayurvedic practices such as self-massage with warm oil (abhyanga) to support circulation, nourish your skin, and promote relaxation.

Chapter 12

Integrating Ayurveda into Modern Life

Despite its ancient roots, Ayurveda can easily be integrated into our fast-paced modern lives.

As we navigate the hustle and bustle of modern life, Ayurveda serves as a gentle guide, nudging us towards a more intentional and mindful approach to living. Whether it's through simple daily practices, nourishing food choices, or personalized self-care rituals, Ayurveda empowers us to create a life that is deeply rooted in our own unique rhythms and needs.

Challenges and Solutions: Common Obstacles in Adopting Ayurveda and How to Overcome Them

Despite its long-standing history and proven effectiveness, Ayurveda faces several challenges in gaining mainstream acceptance and adoption. Let's take a closer look at some of the common obstacles and how we can tackle them head-on.

Common Challenges in Adopting Ayurveda

- **Lack of Awareness and Understanding:** Many people are unfamiliar with Ayurveda and its principles, leading to misconceptions and a reluctance to explore its benefits. For example, some individuals may dismiss Ayurveda as pseudoscience due to a lack of understanding about its holistic approach to healing.

- **Limited Access to Qualified Practitioners:** Finding experienced and well-trained Ayurvedic practitioners can be challenging, especially in certain regions where Ayurveda is not as prevalent. In rural areas or countries where Ayurveda is not widely practiced, individuals may struggle to access reputable practitioners for guidance and treatment.

- **Integration with Modern Medicine:** Many individuals are hesitant to embrace Ayurveda as a standalone treatment due to concerns about its compatibility with modern medical practices. Some doctors may discourage patients from incorporating Ayurvedic remedies alongside conventional treatments, leading to confusion and hesitation.

- **Perception of Ayurveda as Time-Consuming:** The holistic nature of Ayurveda, which emphasizes personalized treatments and lifestyle modifications, may be perceived as requiring significant time and commitment. For example, busy people may struggle to incorporate Ayurvedic practices into their daily routines, viewing it as an additional burden.

Now we know the potential issues, how can we overcome them? Luckily, there are plenty of ways.

Creative Solutions to Overcome Challenges

- **Education and Awareness Campaigns:** Engage in educational initiatives to raise awareness about Ayurveda's benefits and debunk myths surrounding the practice. Host workshops, seminars, and online webinars to provide accessible information to a wider audience.

- **Training and Certification Programs:** Establish training programs for aspiring Ayurvedic practitioners to ensure a steady supply of qualified professionals. Encourage universities and healthcare institutions to offer courses on Ayurveda to increase the expertise and availability of practitioners.

- **Collaboration with Modern Medicine:** Foster partnerships between Ayurvedic and allopathic healthcare providers to create integrated treatment plans for patients. Conduct research studies to validate the efficacy of Ayurvedic practices and build credibility within the medical community.

- **Personalized Ayurvedic Consultations:** Offer online consultations and telehealth services to make Ayurvedic guidance more accessible to individuals with limited access to practitioners. Provide tailored treatment plans and lifestyle recommendations based on each individual's unique constitution and health goals.

By implementing these creative solutions, we can address the challenges hindering the widespread adoption of Ayurveda and pave the way for a more integrated and holistic approach to healthcare.

Combining Ayurveda with Other Health Practices: Finding a Balance with Modern Medicine

In a world where health trends come and go, the timeless wisdom of Ayurveda has stood the test of time, offering holistic and natural solutions to maintain wellness. Combining Ayurveda with modern medicine presents a dynamic approach that harnesses the strengths of both systems to address the complexities of health in the 21st century. It might seem complicated, but it can be done!

The Synergy Between Ayurveda and Modern Medicine

Ayurveda, with its emphasis on balancing mind, body, and spirit, can complement the disease-centric focus of modern medicine by addressing root causes and promoting overall well-being. Then, modern medicine, with its advanced diagnostics and treatments, can provide immediate relief for acute conditions, while Ayurveda focuses on preventive strategies and lifestyle modifications.

For example, a patient with diabetes may benefit from the combination of Ayurvedic dietary recommendations and herbs to regulate blood sugar levels, along with modern medications and monitoring for optimal control. Additionally, yoga and meditation can be incorporated as part of the treatment plan to reduce stress and improve overall health outcomes.

Finding a Balance in Treatment Approaches

Collaborative healthcare teams consisting of Ayurvedic practitioners, modern medicine doctors, nutritionists, and mental health professionals can offer a comprehensive approach to patient care. However, open communication and mutual respect between practitioners of different modalities are key to ensuring a seamless integration of treatments.

Incorporating Ayurvedic Practices in Modern Healthcare Settings

Integrative medicine clinics that offer a range of services from Ayurveda, acupuncture, naturopathy, and modern medicine are gaining popularity as patients seek holistic approaches to health. Wellness retreats and spas that incorporate Ayurvedic principles alongside modern amenities provide a relaxing environment for individuals to rejuvenate and restore balance.

Benefits of Combining Ayurveda with Other Health Practices

There are several benefits of choosing to combine the ancient wisdom of Ayurveda with modern health practices, including:

- **Individualized care:** Ayurveda's focus on understanding each person's unique constitution can enhance personalized treatment plans in conjunction with modern medical interventions.
- **Holistic approach:** By addressing physical, mental, and emotional aspects of health, the integration of Ayurveda with modern medicine can lead to comprehensive healing and improved overall well-being.

But, of course, it doesn't come without its challenges. A lack of standardization and regulation in the Ayurvedic industry can lead to discrepancies in treatment approaches. Seeking qualified and certified practitioners can help ensure quality care. Of course, bridging the gap in knowledge and understanding between Ayurveda and modern medicine through collaborative research and continuing education programs can foster a cohesive approach to healthcare too.

In the end, embracing the strengths of both systems and finding a harmonious balance means we can embark on a journey towards optimal health and wellness that is as unique as we are. Remember, a blend of ancient wisdom and contemporary advancements can pave the way for a healthier and happier you!

Community and Resources: Finding Support and Further Learning

If you've read this far and you're keen to deepen your understanding of Ayurveda and connect with like-minded individuals who share your passion for holistic wellness, you're in luck! Ayurveda is not just a system of medicine; it's a way of life that thrives on community and resources to support its practitioners in their wellness journey.

Importance of Community in Ayurveda

Community plays a vital role in Ayurveda as it provides a supportive environment for individuals to learn, grow, and share their experiences.

Here are some key reasons why community is essential in Ayurveda:

- **Sharing Knowledge and Experiences:** The beauty of Ayurveda lies in its ancient wisdom passed down through generations. By being part of a community of Ayurvedic practitioners and enthusiasts, you can exchange valuable knowledge, tips, and experiences to enhance your understanding of Ayurveda.
- **Accountability and Motivation:** It's easy to veer off track when embarking on a new wellness journey. Being part of a supportive community can help you stay accountable and motivated to follow through with your Ayurvedic practices and lifestyle changes.
- **Emotional Support:** Wellness is not just about physical health; it encompasses mental and emotional well-being as well. Being part of a community allows you to receive emotional support, share your struggles, and celebrate your successes with like-minded individuals.
- **Networking Opportunities:** In the world of Ayurveda, networking is key to expanding your knowledge and growing your practice. By connecting with other practitioners, teachers, and enthusiasts, you open doors to new opportunities for learning and collaboration.

Key Resources for Further Learning in Ayurveda

Now that you understand the importance of community in Ayurveda, let's dive into some key resources that can help you further your learning and connect with like-minded individuals:

- **Ayurvedic Institutes and Schools:** Joining an Ayurvedic institute or school is a great way to immerse yourself in the teachings of Ayurveda. These institutions offer courses, workshops, and training programs led by experienced practitioners and educators.

- **Online Communities and Forums:** In this digital age, online communities and forums provide a convenient platform for connecting with Ayurvedic enthusiasts from around the world. Platforms like Reddit, Facebook groups, and dedicated Ayurveda forums offer a space to ask questions, share resources, and engage in discussions on various Ayurvedic topics.

- **Ayurvedic Retreats and Workshops:** Retreats and workshops offer a unique opportunity to deepen your understanding of Ayurveda in a retreat-style setting. These immersive experiences often include lectures, hands-on workshops, yoga sessions, and Ayurvedic treatments, providing a holistic approach to learning.

- **Ayurvedic Practitioners and Mentors:** Building a relationship with an experienced Ayurvedic practitioner or mentor can provide invaluable guidance and support on your Ayurvedic journey. Look for practitioners who resonate with you and offer mentorship programs or one-on-one consultations.

- **Ayurvedic Books and Publications:** Reading books authored by renowned Ayurvedic experts is a great way to expand your knowledge and explore different perspectives within the field. Some must-read books include "The Complete Book of Ayurvedic Home Remedies" by Vasant Lad and "Ayurveda: The Science of Self-Healing" by Dr. Vasant Lad.

Practical Tips for Finding Support in Ayurveda

Now that you're equipped with knowledge about the importance of community in Ayurveda and key resources for further learning, here are some practical tips for finding the support you need to thrive in your Ayurvedic lifestyle:

- **Attend Ayurvedic Events and Gatherings:** Keep an eye out for Ayurvedic events, workshops, and gatherings in your local community or online. These events offer an opportunity to meet like-minded individuals, learn from experts, and connect with practitioners in your area.

- **Join Online Ayurvedic Groups:** Explore online Ayurvedic groups and communities on social media platforms and forums. Engage in discussions, ask questions, and share your experiences to foster connections with fellow Ayurvedic enthusiasts.
- **Seek Out Local Ayurvedic Practitioners:** Research Ayurvedic practitioners in your area and reach out to them for guidance and support. Many practitioners offer consultations, workshops, and classes that can help you deepen your understanding of Ayurveda and receive personalized recommendations.
- **Start Your Own Ayurvedic Study Group:** Take the initiative to start a study group with friends, family, or colleagues who are interested in Ayurveda. Meet regularly to discuss Ayurvedic concepts, share resources, and support each other on your wellness journey.
- **Invest in Continued Education:** Consider enrolling in advanced courses, workshops, or retreats to further your education in Ayurveda. Investing in continued education not only expands your knowledge but also provides an opportunity to connect with experts and practitioners in the field.
- **Practice Self-Care and Mindfulness:** Remember that self-care and mindfulness are essential components of Ayurveda. Prioritize practices such as meditation, yoga, healthy eating, and adequate rest to support

your overall well-being and stay grounded in your Ayurvedic lifestyle.

Remember, the journey to optimal health is not meant to be taken alone, so embrace the power of community and resources in Ayurveda to enrich your wellness experience!

Personal Stories and Testimonials

It always helps to read real-life stories to give extra weight to the effectiveness of something. When it comes to Ayurveda, there are plenty of real-life experiences to back it up. There are five personal stories and testimonials showcasing the wonderful impact of Ayurveda.

Sarah's Journey to Wellness

Meet Sarah, a busy professional juggling work and family life. Stressed and exhausted, she turned to Ayurveda for balance. Through personalized consultations and dietary changes, Sarah learned to listen to her body. With the help of meditation and herbal supplements, she reclaimed her energy and peace of mind.

Now, Sarah starts her day with yoga and a warm cup of herbal tea, feeling vibrant and centered.

John's Transformation Through Ayurvedic Diet

John struggled with digestive issues for years. Traditional medicine offered little relief until he discovered

Ayurveda. By incorporating digestive spices, like ginger and turmeric, into his meals and following his body's natural rhythms, John found great comfort and healing.

Today, he enthusiastically shares his love for Ayurvedic cooking, inspiring friends and family to embrace the power of food as medicine.

Mia's Ayurvedic Skincare Success

Mia, a skincare enthusiast, battled with stubborn acne for years. Frustrated with chemical-laden products, she sought an alternative in Ayurveda. With the guidance of an Ayurvedic practitioner, Mia adopted a holistic skincare routine using natural ingredients like neem and aloe vera.

Over time, her skin cleared up, revealing a radiant glow. Now, Mia swears by Ayurvedic beauty rituals and encourages others to embrace their natural beauty.

Miguel's Mind-Body Harmony with Ayurvedic Practices

Miguel, a fitness enthusiast, found himself mentally drained despite his rigorous workout routine. Desiring a deeper connection between mind and body, he turned to Ayurveda for guidance. By incorporating daily self-care practices such as oil pulling, tongue scraping, and Abhyanga massage, Miguel experienced a profound shift in his overall well-being.

Today, he exudes vitality and balance, becoming a living testament to the transformative power of Ayurveda.

Lily's Ayurvedic Pregnancy Journey

Lily, a soon-to-be mother, embraced Ayurveda during her pregnancy for a holistic approach to health. Through mindful eating, gentle yoga, and Ayurvedic herbs, she navigated each trimester with grace and ease.

With the support of an Ayurvedic practitioner, Lily experienced a smooth delivery and postpartum recovery. Now, she cherishes the bond she's formed with her baby, grateful for the nourishing principles of Ayurveda that guided her throughout this miraculous journey.

Each of these stories exemplifies the diverse ways in which Ayurveda can positively impact individuals' lives, from enhancing physical wellness to fostering emotional balance.

Through these personal anecdotes, we witness the transformative power of Ayurveda in bringing harmony to mind, body, and spirit. It truly is a holistic approach to well-being that resonates with the essence of who we are.

Conclusion

Now that we're at the end of this book, how are you feeling about introducing Ayurveda into your life? This centuries-old wisdom guides us towards a harmonious balance of mind, body, and spirit. Incorporating its key aspects and practices into your life could be a real game-changer.

But of course, first, you need to be sure that you understand everything about it. That's what this book aims to do. So, before we say goodbye, let's recap the key points we've explored and offer some uplifting words of encouragement for the transformative journey that lies ahead.

Ayurveda, known as the "Science of Life," emphasizes the interconnectedness of all aspects of our being. It recognizes that each individual is unique and requires a personalized approach to achieve optimal well-being. The fundamental principles of Ayurveda revolve around the three doshas, Vata, Pitta, and Kapha, which govern different bodily functions and characteristics.

Understanding your dominant dosha can help you tailor your lifestyle, diet, and wellness practices to restore balance and vitality.

We have delved into the importance of maintaining a daily routine, or Dinacharya, to align ourselves with the natural rhythms of the day and nurture our bodies with self-care rituals. The concept of Ritucharya highlights the significance of adapting our lifestyle according to the changing seasons to stay in tune with nature.

Ayurveda places great emphasis on the role of diet and nutrition in maintaining good health. By incorporating wholesome and seasonal foods that are suitable for your dosha, you can support your body's innate healing wisdom and prevent imbalances. Alongside dietary choices, Ayurveda promotes the use of herbs, spices, and lifestyle practices such as yoga, meditation, and pranayama to create holistic wellness.

Embarking on a journey towards holistic well-being through Ayurveda can be both exciting and challenging. As you explore the world of Ayurvedic principles and practices, remember to approach this path with compassion, curiosity, and an open heart. It's not about striving for perfection but rather about cultivating awareness and making small, sustainable changes that resonate with your unique constitution.

Conclusion

There will be moments of doubt and setbacks along the way, but remember that each step you take towards embracing Ayurveda in your life is a step towards greater balance and vitality. Allow yourself the grace to learn and grow, recognizing that transformation is a gradual process that unfolds at its own pace. Be patient with yourself and trust in the innate intelligence of your body to guide you towards optimal health and well-being.

Surround yourself with a supportive community of like-minded individuals who share your passion for Ayurveda. Seek out teachers, practitioners, and resources that inspire and empower you on your journey. Share your experiences, ask questions, and celebrate your successes, no matter how small they may seem. Remember that you are not alone on this path, and there is a vast network of individuals who are walking alongside you, cheering you on every step of the way.

As you navigate the intricate pathways of Ayurveda, allow yourself to embrace the ebb and flow of life's rhythms with grace and resilience. Stay attuned to your body's signals, listen to its whispers of wisdom, and honor the innate intelligence that resides within you. Let go of the need for external validation or comparison, and instead, cultivate a deep sense of self-awareness and self-love that forms the foundation of your well-being.

In closing, may this journey into the heart of Ayurveda be a catalyst for profound transformation and self-discovery. May you weave the ancient wisdom of Ayurveda into the fabric of your daily life, creating a tapestry of health, harmony, and happiness. Trust in the power of Ayurveda to illuminate your path and guide you towards a life of balance, vitality, and fulfillment. Remember, the journey is not about reaching a destination but about embracing the beauty of the process and the growth that unfolds along the way.

With a heart full of gratitude and a spirit of adventure, step forward into the vibrant world of Ayurveda, knowing that you are embarking on a journey of self-discovery and healing that has the potential to transform your life in ways you never imagined. Embrace this ancient wisdom with an open mind and a willing spirit, and watch as the sacred teachings of Ayurveda unfurl before you, revealing the profound beauty and power of living in harmony with nature and your true self.

May your journey be filled with light, love, and boundless possibilities.

References

Admin. (2024, January 8). *Ayurveda: A Brief Introduction and guide*. Ayurveda. https://ayurveda.com/ayurveda-a-brief-introduction-and-guide/

Banyan Botanicals. (2024, May 1). *Ayurvedic Diet Library | Recipes, Food Combining, Dosha-Specific Foods*. https://www.banyanbotanicals.com/pages/ayurvedic-diet

Clinic, C. (2024, July 2). *What is Ayurveda and does it work?* Cleveland Clinic. https://health.clevelandclinic.org/what-is-ayurveda

Cpt, K. D. M. R. (2023, September 19). *What are the Ayurveda doshas? Vata, Kapha, and Pitta explained*. Healthline. https://www.healthline.com/nutrition/vata-dosha-pitta-dosha-kapha-dosha

Gudritz, L. (2019, August 13). *What happened when I tried the Ayurvedic diet for a week*. Healthline. https://www.healthline.com/health/food-nutrition/i-tried-the-ayurvedic-diet

Jain, R. (2024, February 19). Ayurveda 101: What are the 3 doshas and how to identify yours. *Arhanta Yoga Ashrams*. https://www.arhantayoga.org/blog/what-is-ayurveda-and-its-principles/?utm_source=google&utm_campaign=19237825864&utm_content=&utm_medium=&gad_source=1&gbraid=0AAAADiB6OrbS_SXjkiCaUhVaOdCaE0Cd&gclid=EAIaIQobChMIqr7LxeCmhwMVLpGDBx2A4whLEAAYAyAAEgIUI_D_BwE

Migala, J. (2024, July 9). *What is the Ayurvedic diet? Ayurvedic cooking for beginners.* EverydayHealth.com. https://www.everydayhealth.com/diet-nutrition/ayurvedic-diet/guide/

Principles of Ayurveda. (2023, May 25). Everest Ayurveda. https://www.everest-ayurveda.com/principles-ayurveda

Pukka. (2020, December 9). *Ayurvedic Dosha | Understand your Dosha Type & Real-Life Examples | Pukka Herbs UK.* Pukka Herbs. https://www.pukkaherbs.com/uk/en/wellbeing-articles/understanding-the-dosha

Rd, R. a. M. (2023, November 14). *What is the Ayurvedic diet? benefits, downsides, and more.* Healthline. https://www.healthline.com/nutrition/ayurvedic-diet

The healing benefits of Ayurvedic massage. (n.d.). https://www.ayurvedacollege.net/blogs/the-healing-benefits-of-ayurvedic-massage

Vishram, A. (2023, October 26). *Ayurvedic Massage: A Complete guide — spa Theory.* Spa Theory. https://www.spatheory.com/spa-theory-wellness-beauty-blog/ayurvedic-massage#:~:text=Ayurvedic%20Massage%20offers%20a%20

References

range,and%20spirit%2C%20promoting%20overall%20wellness.

What are the main fundamental principles of Ayurveda? (n.d.). https://www.mamcbhopal.com/what-are-the-main-fundamental-principles-of-ayurveda.php#:~:text=The%20fundamental%20principles%20of%20Ayurveda,Kapha%20(water%20and%20earth).

Wikipedia contributors. (2024, July 2). *Ayurveda.* Wikipedia. https://en.wikipedia.org/wiki/Ayurveda

Worth, T. (2023, November 23). *Ayurveda: Does it really work?* WebMD. https://www.webmd.com/balance/ayurvedic-treatments

About the Author

Monika Daniel, the founder of www.reikisoulacademy.com, is not just a passionate Reiki Master but also a mother of two daughters. This role has significantly influenced her practice, bringing a wealth of compassion and empathy to her work. Her understanding of the importance of nurturing and caring for oneself and others has been deepened through her motherhood journey and her dedication to holistic healing.

Monika's personal journey into the holistic side of life began in Kho Phangyang, Thailand. This journey, filled with self-discovery and growth, led her to embrace a wide array of healing modalities, with a particular focus on Reiki and energy work. Her studies and experiences have enriched her understanding of the healing potential that lies within each of us, inspiring her to share these transformative practices with others.

Monika's commitment to promoting health and wellness is not just a part of her life, it is her life. She is deeply passionate about healthy living, nutrition, and mindfulness, and she actively incorporates these principles into her daily life and teachings, inspiring others to do the same.

Monika's commitment to holistic healing extends beyond her individual practice. She is not just an organizer of retreats; she is a leader. Her passion and dedication create nurturing spaces for individuals to reconnect with themselves and experience profound healing and transformation. Her leadership in these retreats provides a sanctuary for participants to explore holistic practices, cultivate self-awareness, and embark on personal growth and empowerment journeys, instilling a sense of trust and confidence in her abilities.

With a warm heart and an unwavering commitment to the well-being of others, Monika Daniel continues to inspire and uplift those on their path to health, healing, and holistic living.

She dedicates this book to her darling daughters, Sophia and Holly, and her husband, who has supported her throughout this transformative journey.

www.ingramcontent.com/pod-product-compliance
Ingram Content Group UK Ltd.
Pitfield, Milton Keynes, MK11 3LW, UK
UKHW021431270525
6096UKWH00050B/1320